Public Health in the 21st Century

Medicine & Health
New York

Public Health in the 21st Century

Emotionality of COVID-19. Now and After: The War Against a Virus
Maximiliano E. Korstanj (Editor)
Adrian Scribano, PhD (Editor)
2021. ISBN: 978-1-53619-534-7 (Hardcover)
2021. ISBN: 978-1-53619-557-6 (eBook)

Coronavirus Disease: From Molecular to Clinical Perspectives
Yildiz Dincer, PhD (Editor)
2021. ISBN: 978-1-53619-296-4 (Hardcover)
2021. ISBN: 978-1-53619-311-4 (eBook)

More Prescription for Change: Case Studies for Applications of Strategy and Strategic Intervention in National and International Health Systems in Response to a COVID Pandemic
Laure Paquette
2021. ISBN: 978-1-53619-097-7 (Hardcover)
2021. ISBN: 978-1-53619-163-9 (eBook)

COVID-19 and the Rise of Telemedicine: Benefits and Challenges
Christina B. Willis (Editor)
2021. ISBN: 978-1-53619-081-6 (Softcover)
2021. ISBN: 978-1-53619-201-8 (eBook)

The Importance of Natural Products for Public Health: Thymoquinone, Sulforaphane, Phloretin and Epigallocatechin
Dr. Mohamad Hesam Shahrajabian
Dr. Wenli Sun
Alessandra Paragone
Dr. Qi Cheng
2020. ISBN: 978-1-53618-964-3 (eBook)

More information about this series can be found at https://novapublishers.com/product-category/series/public-health-in-the-21st-century/

Stephen M. Magu, PhD

Barakoa (Mask) During COVID-19

Malevolent Pathogens and Pandemic Responses in Kenya after 600 Days

nova
Medicine & Health
New York

DOI: https://doi.org/10.52305/UEGU1362

Library of Congress Cataloging-in-Publication Data

ISBN: 978-1-68507-798-3

Published by Nova Science Publishers, Inc. † New York

This short volume is dedicated to all those who did everything to survive the 100-year COVID-19 pandemic from 2020 onwards, including those who were infected and subsequently recovered. It is also dedicated to all the brave frontline workers who served their communities at great peril to themselves and their loved ones. It is dedicated to all the scientists who worked tirelessly to find vaccines and therapeutics and ways to deal with the illness.

As always, it is dedicated to the brightest constellation among all the stars in all the galaxies, my mother, Mary W. Magu, who almost religiously sanitized, wore masks and took care of family whose health faltered under a relentless virus.

And, with condolences, to all those who were lost in the pandemic.

Contents

Preface

On January 12th 2020, the premier global institution at the forefront of managing especially global health issues, the World Health Organization (WHO) declared that a new form of a highly contagious, severe acute respiratory syndrome coronavirus 2 (SARS-CoV-2) had been spreading in Wuhan City, Hubei Province in China, since January 2020. Subsequently, new evidence would suggest that perhaps the soon-to-be-pandemic had been spreading much earlier, perhaps as early as October 2019. Despite the tight control of information practiced by the Chinese government on most aspects of the virus, its origins or the earliest diagnoses, control that extended to challenging a specific initial date or even the origins (lab leak or the meat market), as early as December or even November 2019, the illness, now widely referred to as COVID-19, was already infecting individuals in the region and possibly spreading elsewhere in the world. In what often amounted to 'muddying the waters,' there were suggestions that the flu-like illness might have been, even possibly originated in France, or Italy.

It took another nearly 60 days for the WHO to declare the illness a global pandemic, at which point its global spread was barely contained. What would be later termed as 'community spread' across borders, nations and oceans was already underfoot, in most cases, asymptomatically and undetected for anywhere up to a week. The WHO also made clear that, for purposes of uniformity and reducing ambiguity, the new flu would be subjected to the WHO's Emergency Committee on the novel coronavirus (2019-nCoV)'s determination and naming process in order to settle on a preliminary, interim name for the new disease. This led to the selection of the "2019-nCoV acute respiratory disease" – or 2019-nCoV – in line with best practices by the International Classification of Diseases (ICD). Later, a more 'permanent' name was to be selected by WHO's International Committee on Taxonomy of

Viruses (ICTV). The ICTV settled on the less tongue-breaking, less-taxing COVID-19 disease.[1]

Beyond the initial panic, finger-pointing and collective confusion over how to address the new 'flu', leading to some initial, almost drastic overreactions, there was an urgent need to consider the next actions and perhaps mitigation and control strategies. The varied response to COVID-19 around the world became a source of fascination – fascination of the kind where one is a spectator in a morbidly fascinating, terrible and often, a sense of helpless inability to intervene – such as watching an accident in real-time. Some responses were outright violations of individuals and human rights, others were draconian, to say the least. Reactions by governments, as well as their citizens, often brought out the worst in humanity, but also showed the sheer ineptitude of political rather than scientific, medical decisions. Because the virus especially overwhelmed the arguably more prosperous Global North nations, especially Italy, the US and soon, other European nations, the Global South had a bit of time to learn from what worked and what didn't.

What was especially heartbreaking, and what would be repeated in many other countries, was the Italian experience, played out on a free, democratic-society type of openly available information. Seeing doctors clad in the doomsday scenario-type head-to-toe hazmat suits, their patients struggling to breathe and hooked up to space-looking hospital contraptions supplying oxygen, while other individuals were dying alone because hospitals were both death and no-go zones, city squares were emptying and the world-famous Italian peoples' love for wine and pizza on the plaza moved inside was positively frightening. The lockdowns of the northern Italian regions such as Lombardy only produced an inevitable, almost predictable scramble to get out of the soon-to-be locked-down areas. It was predictable – every end-of-times movie with a pandemic motive ends in such scrambles. While the very human response is to get out of the way of danger, it was not clear (nor is it now) that most countries had envisioned lockdowns or evacuations in the event of a hundred-year pandemic. This particular reaction, however, ignored the possibility that the virus was not particularly keen on obeying the *Mona Lisa*, let alone the Lombardy governor. It was even quite likely that the virus was escaping with those fleeing it. Essentially, the initial strategy coming out of Italy would have looked familiar to Sandro Botticelli even as he painted *The Banquet in the Pine Forest* based on Giovanni Boccaccio's *Decameron*.

---

[1] WHO, "Novel Coronavirus (2019-nCoV): Situation Report – 10," *The World Health Organization*, 30 January, 2020, https://www.who.int/docs/default-source/coronaviruse/situation-reports/20200130-sitrep-10-ncov.pdf?sfvrsn=d0b2e480_2.

Soon, the world would learn – from Italians, Europeans, Chinese, health officials and other epidemiologists from across the world – of terms such as Protective Personal Equipment (PPE), social-distancing measures, masks (some with attitude), K-95, surgical masks, sanitizing, lockdowns, serums, seroprevalence, a higher level of awareness of WFH – work from home, Zoom, Collaborate, (self-) quarantines, COVID-19 tests, PCR, remdesivir, empty stadiums, first-responders, home therapy, Johnson & Johnson vaccine, Moderna, Pfizer, Sinovac, even vaccine-skeptics and 'vaccine nationalism.' The planet found a reason to collectively hate medical providers for devising the worst test in human history, one whose design assures that part of the brain is likely scratched during each test. Most of the new terms and their implications came from the west but the rest of the world would soon learn it. The west had a few advantages that potentially supported their mitigation strategies, such as welfare support, expert and robust medical systems, gene-altering scientific research and ability to impose robust travel limits.

Whereas the subject of this short treatise is Kenya's experience with COVID-19, the United Kingdom is an especially informative case study. This is in part because on February 6th, it had a mere three cases (barring widely hypothesized undetected community spread). The UK did not implement any significant public health measures in a timely manner, despite daily, emergent and alarming evidence from continental Europe, especially Italy. Even after the WHO's also widely criticized-as-delayed declaration of a global pandemic, the UK was ambivalent, only taking steps to constrain the sale of medications whose efficacy was suspect.

It was not until the 20th of March that the UK Prime Minister, Boris Johnson, with as much great theatrical flourish as could simultaneously be tempered with the weight of the decision he was making, ordered the closure of those establishments deemed efficient disease vectors, such as clubs and bars, looked in the camera and told Britons to "stay home." By then, it is likely that the Prime Minister was already infected and heading towards his famously near-death experience, one that was said to alter his entire perspective on the pandemic, and which led to accusations of swinging the pendulum too far in the other direction and excessive amounts of caution.

The next few months would evoke the very same spectacle of watching all of the UK's numbers rocket upwards: infections, deaths, the daily appreciations of especially medical workers, and Captain Sir Tom Moore, for walking the garden. The UK's devolved governments took uneven approaches to contain the pandemic, and it wasn't difficult to wonder how ever Britannia ruled the waves given such…challenges, inertia and inability to decisively deal with the pandemic's progress and implications. The importance of other countries' reactions and measures is that other nations co-opted them, or variations thereof.

Kenya was one such country. Its earliest responses mimicked the UK's almost to the letter, although its first case was reported on March 12th, 2020. This was just one day after the US declared COVID-19 a national emergency. Benefitting from evidence from the tragedy and travesty unfolding in Europe, the Kenyan government reacted swiftly and decisively. But beyond that, the practical implementation of curfews and lockdowns seemed unable to escape Finagle's Law of Dynamic Negatives – that *anything that can go wrong, will—at the worst possible moment*. A few days after the first case was diagnosed, Kenya's president Uhuru Kenyatta outlined proposed measures to keep the contagion from spreading. They included restricting travel from countries with confirmed COVID-19 cases, limiting (re)entry into Kenya only to Kenyan citizens and residents, closure of schools, tele-working for government officers, promoting the use of cashless transactions, placing limits on social events (fundraisers, funerals, church meetings), sanitization, disinfection of incoming foreign vessels and crews, their (mandatory) quarantine and the establishment of a toll-free number for all matters related to COVID-19.

This was decidedly aggressive.

The country had a paltry 15 cases by March 22nd *and* was clamping down in ways reminiscent of an autocracy that was the suspected origin, China, rather than as a democracy. Case counts rose slowly, reaching 81 by 1st April. The government's strategies, containment measures and public health policies were meant to limit contagion and eventually hopefully eliminate the pandemic altogether, yet inherent in the totality of its response were structural, administrative, governance, public health emergency mitigation and social policy errors. On the one hand, this was fairly understandable: the country had never dealt with a major pandemic or public health crisis, let alone a hundred-year pandemic. At the same time, every response, while it may have been well intended, appeared to essentially bring out the very possibly worst outcome in application and results.

November 1st, 2021 marked the 600th day that the country was grappling with the COVID-19 pandemic. It is the goal of this short treatise to examine the responses by different sections of the Kenyan society to the COVID-10 pandemic. These include the Kenyan government's response, the citizens' responses, medical professions and the health agency as well as the other stakeholders. It assesses the overall success in dealing with COVID-19.

Preliminaries

Timeline of the COVID-19 Pandemic in Kenya

2020

- March 11th: 1st confirmed COVID-19 case diagnosed in the country
- March 15th: President Uhuru Kenyatta outlined measures to combat the illness, including closure of most government offices for tele-working and closing schools
- March 26th: First COVID-19 death reported
- March 27th: 7 p.m. to 5 a.m. curfew begins; on day 1, Kenyans are whipped and arbitrarily held almost 2 hours before official start; deaths reported
- March 31st: 18 days after the first case was diagnosed, total case count reaches 59
- April 6th: The government imposes a lockdown (ban on movement in and out of four counties: that is Nairobi, Mombasa, and Kilifi and Kwale)
- By mid-April, total tests performed were 2,366; end April: total cases reach 396 with 17 deaths
- 6th June: 7 pm to 4 am curfew extended 30 days, modified to 9 pm to 4 am
- 15th June: one of the last counties to record COVID-19 infections, Nyandarua, still had no cases
- July: the 1st wave's high peak reached, with almost 1,000 daily cases diagnosed end July.
- December: total cases approach 100,000 (96,000+); governor Nyangarama dies from COVID. Second wave now fully afoot; up to 1,600 positive cases per day diagnosed (Source: Ministry of Health, Republic of Kenya)

2021

- January: total case count passes 100,000 with 100,773 diagnosed positive; deaths at 1,770
- March: third wave afoot; up to 2,000 positive cases a day diagnosed March 20th - 31st
- March 26th: New lockdown imposed on movement into and out of five counties: Nairobi, Kajiado, Machakos, Kiambu, and Nakuru. Curfew for these counties modified – from 8:00 pm to 4:00 am
- June 12th: Total Vaccinations administered finally hit 1 million (or 1.89% of the population)
- June 16th: The government imposes new containment measures for 13 counties in Western and Nyanza regions as COVID-19 cases spike again (and totaled 177,000 total cases)
- August, 2021: The government relaxes the social-distancing rule for public transportation; it also accepts a tranche of vaccines from Greece, US and Latvia
- Possible fourth wave in progress, a high of 1,600 cases diagnosed in mid-August
- On September 1, 2021, the Ministry of Health reports 2,850, 932 vaccines having been given; 50,000 shy of 2 million (first dose) and 200,000 shy of 1 million for second doses.

List of Persons, Abbreviations, and Terms

Select COVID-19-Related Key Persons, Groups and Organizations

CS Health:	(Cabinet Secretary for) Health, Mutahi Kagwe
CAS	(Chief Administrative Secretary)
Education CS	(Cabinet Secretary for) Education, George Magoha
Interior CS	(Cabinet Secretary for) Interior and Coordination of Government, Fred Matiang'i
KEMRI	Kenya Medical Research Institute
KEMSA	Kenya Medical Supply Association
NERC	National Emergency Response Committee

Abbreviations of Some Uncommon Terms

COVID-19	Severe acute respiratory syndrome coronavirus 2 (SARS-Cov-2), 2019-nCoV or COVID-19
LHC	'Long-haul COVID-19' (COVID-19 symptoms that linger longer than about 30 days)
PPE	Personal Protective Equipment (includes masks, gloves, face shields, bio-suits and other protective gear to avoid contracting the COVID-19 virus
WFH	Work from Home

COVID-19's New Vocabulary [or Increased Use due to COVID]

Barakoa	(Face) mask or face-covering (swahili translation)
COVID millionaires	Individuals suspected of benefitting from aspects of COVID-19 mitigation and containment in KEMSA's PPE provision and tenders awarded to day-old companies
Mask mandates	requirements imposed by lawful authorities for individuals to wear some form of face covering especially in public and indoors to reduce transmission
Sanitizing	Using soap/disinfectant to clean hands and surfaces that may harbor COVID
Social distance	The practice of observing physical separation of individuals by anywhere from three to six feet (1 – 2 meters) to contain aerosolized droplets' transmission
Wuhan	City of Wuhan in Hebei Province, China, suspected COVID-19 origin
Zoom	Class of video-calls (meetings, etc., carried out online via video teleconnection)
Zoom economy	Increasing use of tele-working across many sectors of most countries' economy

Introduction

In the coming years, perhaps at a scale greater than the 1918 Spanish flu's outcomes, tomes will be written, intent on dissecting the various elements of the SARS-COV-2 virus and the COVID-19 pandemic. Even museums, which have taken to chronicling the progress (or lack thereof) of COVID-19 in real-time, will contribute to these debates. At the height of the pandemic, its various aspects dominated almost every major news conference, most legislation, even disagreements but especially individuals' lives. Mankind would soon begin go learn about 'mutations,' with each appearing to be more dire than the next: the British – B.1.1.7 variant, the South African variant, the Brazilian strain and most recently, what was considered one of the most contagious and devastating, India-originating Delta variant, quickly followed by the rapidly-transmitting, shorter incubating Omicron variant, with its subsequent B.2 variant and even more recently, a possible 'deltacron' variant.

Evidence of the changes in our awareness of the COVID-19 pandemic was procured in the form of the previously innocuous scientists holding positions such as the Director of the National Institute of Allergy and Infectious Diseases (NIAID) and the Chief Medical Advisor to the President, the CDC director, the Surgeon General of the United States, the FDA Administrator, the Director of the WHO and even Kenya's Director General for Health becoming well known and highly visible. They began dominating conferences, TV appearances, briefings and even global meetings. Even as the science (and virus) evolved, sometimes frustratingly, the world looked to these very people to find answers to the pandemic. These ranged from the origins of the virus to its avenues for transmission to the most effective vaccines to the length of coverage and immunity one gets from the vaccine. At the same time, each of their new finds ended with the cautious, very worrisome statement, that 'we are still learning about this virus,' particularly when it mutates.

Luckily, human beings learn, and the past year-plus has seen us learn (or not), sometimes quickly, raising hope that perhaps mankind might still survive. But man also knows that he knows some things. Collectively, we don't know that we know everything there is to know about the virus, its origin, its development into a global pandemic, the mutations that seem to adapt better than previous variants and transmit with extinction-level lethality, whether the safe non-transmission distance is three feet or six feet, on surfaces or if planes are safer than grocery stores and supermarkets, the virus' own DNA, COVID-19 cures and other things. Indeed, when one considers everything we know, it is possible that there is much we still don't know we don't know. The recently deceased, controversial but oft-quoted Donald Rumsfeld may not have intended to sound Socratic, but COVID-19 has levels of fluid lethality that might only present in hot lava.

Still, there are those elements of our growing understanding of the virus and the pandemic and governmental responses that, over a year and a half later, can be evaluated and their success, or lack thereof, considered. They include responses by governments, citizens, scientists, and other actors, including the virus itself. In particular, were there actual aliens studying the collective human response to a virus that affects people mostly the same way, one such alien might be tempted to wonder why there are varying responses by different countries and authorities, or even belief levels about whether the virus exists or is as lethal as suggested. There is not a universal global response to a virus that respects no borders, fears no tweets, likely celebrates denials of its existence, and has no respect for presidential exhortations not to fear COVID-19.[2]

The goal of this treatise then, is to attempt a systematic examination of Kenya's responses to COVID-19. As noted, Kenya's first case was identified on March 11th, 2020. Four days later, on March 15th, in an agenda-setting, much awaited prime-time address to the nation, Uhuru Kenyatta, the president, outlined government measures to combat COVID-19 illness. These included the immediate closure of most government offices and businesses being encouraged to implement tele-working, and the closing of schools, churches, mosques and other events where Kenyans congregated.[3] There would be curfews, bans on movement, partial lockdowns and sanitizing – there would also be limited help by the government, especially to those deemed most vulnerable, actions that were somewhat insufficient.

---

[2] Christian Paz, "All the President's Lies About the Coronavirus," *The Atlantic - Politics*, Updated at 2:20 p.m. ET on November 2, 2020. https://www.theatlantic.com/politics/archive/2020/11/trumps-lies-about-coronavirus/608647/.

[3] Presidential Strategic Communication Unit (PSCU). *Address to the Nation by H.E. Uhuru Kenyatta on COVID-19 [...]* 15th March 2020. (Web). URL: https://www.president.go.ke/2020/03/15/.

A year later, in an address commemorating the first anniversary of the first COVID-19 case, the presidential address took stock of COVID-19's tally: 1,879 deaths, more than 100,000 infections, almost 1.4 million tests administered, and half a million vaccine doses in a population of 53 million as of April 14th, 2021. It was clear that the country was not out of the woods yet, and was, indeed, on the cusp of a third wave. It should not have come as a surprise: it has never been clear that the virus stopped spreading after 10 p.m., or 7 p.m., and Kenya's half-hearted measures were as frustrating as they were ineffective as is increasingly clear. Indeed, one could have been easily forgiven if they argued that throughout the pandemic, the government has lacked clear, cohesive strategies, and has almost lurched from one 'hope' to another.

By the same year-mark, other numbers were anything but comforting: from a projected annual economic growth of 6.2% for 2020, the country's economy grew by only 0.6%, and many citizens were estimated to have fallen into poverty. The pandemic's highest positivity rate was witnessed in November 2020 at 19%. That it had climbed back up to 13% in March 2021, before dipping to 10% in June 2021 (on another projected rise) illustrates the very definition of the start of waves on waves.[4] Kenya's COVID-19 testing regime, comparable to that of most other African countries, has been abysmal, with an average of 5,000 tests carried out daily on a population of 54 million and which, surprisingly, has produced 3.36 million tests and 323,000 infections, against a total of 16.5 million vaccine doses administered.

For the tests, the figure computes to a high of 0.17 tests per thousand and even with the higher 3.6 million number, to 6.22% of the citizens tested. In comparison, during the same period, the number of COVID-19 tests per thousand performed in the US came to 5.63 long before government even started shipping tests to households. As of July 2021, US tests were outpacing Kenya's by a factor of 33. South Africa was tripling Kenya's number during the same period. Ultimately, the US' total of 410 million tests by early April 2021 outstripped Kenya's 1.6 million by a factor of 256.[5] In the second year of the pandemic, around July and August 2021, the number of tests marginally went up to about 10,000 a day. But even then, it has never been clear whether

---

[4] Presidential Strategic Communication Unit (PSCU). *The Fourteenth [14th] Presidential Address on the Coronavirus Pandemic.* Friday 12th March, 2021 (Web). URL: https://www.president.go.ke/2021/03/12.

[5] Hannah Ritchie, Esteban Ortiz-Ospina, Diana Beltekian, Edouard Mathieu, Joe Hasell, Bobbie Macdonald, Charlie Giattino and Cameron Appel, "Coronavirus (COVID-19) Testing," *Our World in Data*, (Web), updated April 9, 2021. URL: https://ourworldindata.org/coronavirus-testing#how-many-tests-are-performed-each-day.

these include the tests that are performed on individuals who need to travel, or whether it is those carried out in hospitals when citizens go for treatment when they are unwell, particularly absent mass-testing. One wonders then, whether even the positivity rate was ever accurate, given the low number of tests performed.

A deeper dive into Kenya's other responses is a study in head-scratching contrasts. When the first COVID-19 case was reported on March 12th 2020, the very same day the US declared a national emergency, Kenya prepared to implement mitigation strategies, with the benefit of evidence and lesions from the tragedy that was unfolding in Europe. The proposed mitigation strategy announced on 15th March included restricting travel from countries with COVID-19 cases, limiting re-entry to Kenyan citizens and residents, mandatory 14-day quarantine for all arrivals within the previous 2 weeks, school closure (primary and secondary) and Higher Education Institutions, tele-working for government officers and private businesses when possible, cashless transactions, limiting social events, encouraging businesses to provide sanitization resources, disinfecting incoming foreign vessels and crews including a (mandatory) quarantine and a toll-free number for public reporting on COVID-19-related matters. By March 22nd, the country had recorded a paltry 15 cases by March 22, reaching 81 by 1st April, 2020.

Kenya's responses to COVID-19 have been puzzling, inconsistent, inadequate and altogether led to less-than-optimum outcomes in the COVID-19 fight. Within the first month of the first case being diagnosed, more people died at the hands of police enforcing curfews than did from the virus itself. Since then, mitigation actions have included an increase in opportunities for more rent-seeking (at every level, from government bureaucratic corruption and one-day billionaires to local enforcement levels), executive mismanagement and inconsistency, public skepticism of the pandemic itself and the potential impact of the public health measures and a glaring lack of consultation of all stakeholders.

A further trend evident everywhere around the world and labeled here as 'political' non-compliance with public health measures has been persistent, where elites flout public health guidelines to carry out political activities. For citizens, economic distress is evident; it has impacted compliance with social distancing, curfews and the ban on movement that potentially leads to transmission. Even for those that die of COVID-19, the proposal to continue the observance of socio-cultural traditions that imperil any potential progress in combating the pandemic are always evident, such as burial rites and life celebrations. There has been a lot of 'magical thinking,' including religiously inspired spiritual explanations, exemptions, proposed cures and especially egregiously and poor public compliance in the religious settings. Peculiar to Kenya, most 'compliance' is done to avoid arrest and the Kshs. 500 fine, rather than from the belief that such measures aid public health and control of COVID-19.

The objective of this research project is to i) evaluate the progress of the pandemic, ii) assess the governmental, public and private institutional mitigation strategies for COVID-19, iii) interrogate government responses and programs to reduce public interactions (such as the practicability of social distancing in public transport, income support, distribution of food aid) and iv) the level of preparation of Kenya's infrastructure (from transport to electrical grid to internet access in order to access at-home services – from schooling to recovery), and v) lessons from COVID-19 to future health crises, but also to prepare for efficiency in conducting business in the context of limited in-person interactions.

To evaluate these issues and consider their impacts on the level of success – or not – that Kenya has achieved in the first 600 days of the pandemic, the research examines the responses through several lenses. They are divided roughly into broad categories and several sub-categories. They especially focus on planning and government responses (administrative, public health, economic and institutional), socio-cultural responses (religion, cultural traditions, and social welfare responses); the mitigation's outcomes (wellness, food and nutrition, government and governance, security, education and human development), and the unintended consequences of the pandemic on society more broadly, such as corruption and new avenues of such activity.

Other sources of evaluation of overall responses point to key government enforcement actions and responses that are more widespread, and include keen surveillance over travel and travelers, quarantines, curfews, closing facilities such as schools, limiting immigration, epidemiological responses (use of PPE, public health guidance on masks, hand-washing and social distancing, home recovery, burial windows for COVID-19 victims and designation of COVID-19 hospitals) and welfare responses or lack thereof. It also considers the social, cultural and religious responses (for example, weddings, religious services, burial ceremonies, traditions and superstitions in line with African traditions).

There have been other 'miscellaneous' responses and outcomes: they include (im)proper use of masks (hanging around the chin), nutritional and educational challenges, increasing poverty and the difficulty of care imposed by multi-generational households impacting the proposed home recovery without spreading the pandemic, exclusion experienced by individuals diagnosed with COVID-19 among others. Of special note are the unintended consequences of government responses, classified here as 'negative responses' (corruption and non-social distancing in public transport upon payment of a bribe, improperly procured PPE and the question of how World Bank funding, comprising of an initial US$60 Million (KSh6.1 billion) in March 2020 and a further US$1 Billion in May 2020, for a total of Kshs. 106 billion, was allocated), and the impact of the proposed Building Bridges Initiatives (BBI) aimed at securing a referendum to modify the constitution.

Structure of the Book

This brief account employs an analysis of proposals and policies that the government has enacted at the various levels – policies it has attempted to implement and the success thereof. It also examines citizens' responses solicited through observation and informal interviews, scrutiny of chats on streaming content covering Kenya's responses, and aggregates various other submissions solicited through social media. The essential goal is to combine both government and citizens' perspectives as to the most significant issues that have surrounded the pandemic, the perception of their effectiveness, the impacts on individuals and society, and mitigation measures across the country and citizens' sense of government's ability to address the pandemic and its effects.

As important as participatory research is and can be, one recognizes too, that citizens' perceptions and perspectives may be influenced by a variety of factors, and therefore, does not necessarily make these responses utilitarian or well-informed. Indeed, evidence from other areas and countries, including those with more, better access to information, has shown high levels of skepticism, hesitancy and consumption of misinformation. Notwithstanding, in the first section, the research addresses the wholesome government responses beginning with the early days of the pandemic, including curfews, movement cessation and other mitigation strategies. Government responses can be broadly classified under a number of sub-headings: there were different types of fiscal, security-related, administrative and public health, to name but a few.

By themselves, the public health responses, driven by scientific research, global best practices and recommendations by the likes of KEMRI, were instrumental in informing the actions and reactions by the citizenry as directed (or not) by the government, sometimes haphazardly. As such, government's actions and responses should be considered first, followed by the different reactions to the guidance and positions, and the occasional modifications to the guidance. These following sections attempt to lay out, and where possible, assess government responses: how many curfews, where, when why and even whether or not they have been effective. The account then goes on to consider the impact of the strategies and responses, especially with reference to the regular citizen. There were socio-cultural outcomes and impacts, which are as important, perhaps more so than the economic, but also human resource, education-related impacts that have confounded all and sundry.

Evidently, because the pandemic keeps ebbing and flowing, not just in Kenya, but also in the other parts of the world *including those previously reporting high testing, mask usage and vaccination rates,* the assessment of the strategies, the impacts and citizens' reactions to the currently ongoing COVID-19 pandemic must, of necessity, be functionally incomplete and only partial. This treatise concedes as much. When the final story of the pandemic is written many years into the future, this volume might only account for a slim part of the story that will be told to future Kenyans – or whichever nationality they might *then* assume. Readers ought to keep in mind that this writing aims to correspond with the 600th day of Kenya's experience with and response to the COVID-19 pandemic, and thus is not necessarily a complete and full account of how Kenya's government has dealt with the COVID-19 pandemic, which is in some instances being now considered endemic, rather than strictly a pandemic.

Chapter 1

The Kenyan Government's COVID-19 Administrative Responses and Strategies

Abstract

This chapter examines some of the more macro processes of managing the pandemic as they have been implemented by the Kenyan government to date. They include the issues related to official communication, provision of public information and consistent messaging, the role of the various government institutions in the (mis)communication, public information on such issues as lock-downs, vaccines (their availability, brands and safety) and institutional disaster management as part of government response. It also examines the role of government in stopping (or facilitating limited) movement (travel bans, lockdowns etc., and how government communicated these), the inequality produced by the pandemic and the interplay of the Kenyan government's relations with and reactions to other nations in the management of the pandemic in the country particularly where interstate trade is occurring (here, the discussion specifically focuses on Tanzania, an early COVID-19 'skeptic) and its decisions' impacts on Kenya. Some of the selected sub-topics covered here include: government communications, public information and emergency management; communication (and) messaging; public information and communications: (with) various public and private institutions as collaborators or non-cooperating entities; production and delivery of public information and the government's communications on vaccines; institutional disaster and pandemic management: government by committee – NERC; human movement: transmission; constraining human movement: curfews, lockdowns and travel bans; COVID curfews and pandemic inequality; and COVID-Complexity: Tanzania's COVID-19 denials and impacts.

Novel Pandemic, Suspect Capacity and Steep Learning Curves

Like many other countries around the world, the Kenyan government sought to contain the spread, and mitigate the impacts that COVID-19 would undoubtedly bring to the country and its people. While the difficulties of having a long border might be enviable because it implies 'big;' having many neighbors in the age of COVID-19 brought uncovered the challenges of managing human movement in a nuanced way to assure their livelihoods *and* contain the pandemic. Kenya has quite a substantive border, which stretches approximately 3,457km (2,160 mi) and five land neighbors.[6]

On each of its borders, there are ethnically related groups living on different sides, frequently interacting with little constraint and giving life to the well-worn, but somewhat disputed 'six degrees of separation.'[7] These are groups that, despite the existence of internationally recognized borders, have lived next to each other for millennia, trading, intermarrying, carrying on the business of neighbors and occasionally, even conducting war. They are highly interconnected; their interconnectedness, and hence any attempts at separating them, even during a pandemic such as COVID-19, challenges governments and their policing of borders. COVID-19's transmission leaves little room for error regarding measures to contain its spread. This was especially the case when two, or more countries operated on the basis of differing levels of COVID-19 threat assessment, belief or disbelief, as did countries all over the world. For Madagascar, and island, this had little impact. For Kenya, its southern neighbor's decision not to take COVID-19 seriously illuminated challenges that would soon challenge its own strategies and approaches that were well-tested and working elsewhere. As the war against COVID-19, some of Kenya's viable tools would be rendered useless due to Tanzania's actions. President Uhuru Kenyatta's government's initial plans have been outlined elsewhere in this chapter. These include the initial, nationally-televised speech on March 15th 2020 and the major steps the government had determined to be most critical in preventing the spread. Still, it is useful to re-consider them in a systematic way, especially from governmental and administrative perspectives; their implementation, their effects, and an assessment of their effectiveness. One might suggest that examining the epidemiological and public health measures and outcomes might be more useful, but since some of these were directed by government actions, their implementation is most profitably contemplated under the umbrella of the government's administrative actions and related responses.

---

[6] CIA, "Kenya," *The World Factbook*, Page last updated: June 29, 2021, https://www.cia.gov/the-world-factbook/countries/kenya/.

[7] Stanley Milgram, "The Small World Problem," *Psychology Today*, vol. 1, no. 1 (May 1967), 61-66.

Government Communications, Public Information and Emergency Management

By the time COVID-19 came bursting onto the global scene between December 2019 and January 2020, public information and communication in the digital and information age was already undergoing major, interesting and in some instances, destructive changes, even assault. As of January 2021, the Washington Post estimated that the-then US president had "accumulated 30,573 untruths,"[8] a dressed-up term for 'lies;' this came to about 21 'erroneous claims' a day. Information that did not correlate with a preferred, mostly self-serving point of view became 'fake news.' Coming from the top levels of (any) government, potential for erosion of confidence in the same government including public health measures existed, and in the course of COVID-19 management there and in countries like Brazil and Tanzania became impossible.

To further illustrate the role that information has played especially within the timeframe that Kenya's COVID-19 responses are considered, it is useful to consider the origins of SARS-CoV-2, the virus that causes COVID-19. Suspicions have been advanced, that the virus came from the Wuhan Institute of Virology (or Wuhan Lab, or elsewhere), that the virus was engineered by humans, or that it possibly jumped from bats, pangolins and other animals onto humans. Going on two years later, it is not clear what the source was. Other elements of the pandemic are also hotly contested: for example, whether the vaccines transmit live virus, whether they are safe, or cause infertility, or whether Bill Gates is implanting people with trackers. Although these possibilities are scientifically far-fetched, the kind of information available raises a broader question of whether truth is possible and – or relative. Although this is a discussion for a different time and place, if one considers Rational Choice Theory (RCT) and its premises as having merit, nothing is more important than the correct information.

Access to information has gradually evolved, especially in the information age and such concepts as Internet of Things (IoT). Information is available at the speed of Alexa or Siri, but so is misinformation. Governments, except perhaps those of China, North Korea and other countries not considered democratic and therefore constraining free access to information (or

---

[8] Glenn Kessler, Salvador Rizzo and Meg Kelly, "Trump's false or misleading claims total 30,573 over 4 years," The *Washington Post - Fact Checker*, Jan. 24, 2021, https://www.washingtonpost.com/politics/2021/01/24/trumps-false-or-misleading-claims-total-30573-over-four-years/.

misinformation), no longer have the monopoly over what the public knows. Most cell phones today are essentially carried by journalists-in-motion. Facebook's 'population,' with over 2.85 billion monthly active users, is greater than India and China's combined, and a marketplace of good and bad ideas, theories and conspiracies, as well as accurate information. Of its total users, almost 9 million are in Kenya; their ability to share (mis)information is further assisted by the free data available to Facebook, Messenger and WhatsApp. In this kind of environment, government has had to be especially active to provide - accurate - information, debunk myths, negate rumors, promote COVID-19 mitigation strategies, vaccines and other good practices.

In the initial stages of COVID-19 in Kenya, near-daily briefings, especially by the Ministry of Health's top officials including the CS (Hon. Mũtahi Kagwe), the Health Director General (Dr. Patrick Amoth) and the Chief Administrative Secretary (Dr. Mercy Mwangangi) were permanent fixtures in front of cameras. They needed to be; rumors over every aspect of the pandemic, including the transmission, were rife and needed countering. Besides the Ministry of Health, other especially important briefings and statements issued from members of the NERC, including the Education CS, and the CS Interior (who also held the portfolio of coordination of government).

To the extent that these public briefings were held, citizens had access to accurate information in a timely fashion, though the level of access to means of information (such as TV and newspapers, as measured through the Globalization Index),[9] remains far below comparable countries around the world even with a 100.3% mobile penetration rate. The coordination and collaboration with private media, including some of the biggest media houses such as Nation Media, Standard Media, Kenya Broadcasting Corporation and even vernacular radio and TV stations facilitated access to official channels of information, government policy and strategies, although it is not clear that this necessarily curtailed the rather creative imagination license that most Kenyans afford themselves.

[9] Savina Gygli, Florian Haelg, Niklas Potrafke and Jan-Egbert Sturm, "The KOF Globalisation Index – Revisited," *Review of International Organizations,* Vol. 14, No. 3, (2019), 543-574 https://doi.org/10.1007/s11558-019-09344-2.

Communication: Messaging

Having the tools to communicate does not necessarily mean that one is communicating, and providing the right information does not mean that it is reaching the intended audience or that it is understood as intended. As critical as the daily and occasional briefings have been as the country and the world go, or went through steep learning curves, opportunities were missed, rumors spread, misperceptions were not addressed and the wildfire that is gossip took hold, spurred on by tools of modern communication, especially Facebook, WhatsApp and Twitter and free data. In Kenya, one of the most significant and impactful failures in communication was in failing to change the perception of COVID-19: from origin to arrival in the country, and especially emphasizing its universal transmissibility to and by anyone with lungs. This led to shunning some of the earliest patients, even from patients' own families.

As it spread in early March and caused great disruption across all spheres, COVID-19 was approached, and treated more like HIV-AIDS and its reputation mirrored the latter's in the 1990s: and it was one of exclusion. Messages communicated by the government clarifying that COVID-19's aerosolized transmission made it capable of infecting any and all who had lungs, and breathed, hence *all* Kenyans were potential targets for infection, might have helped (slightly) change this perception. However, government strategies and actions to set up several isolation, quarantine and treatment facilities that were built around Level 5 hospitals in different counties, Nyayo Wards and other 'Referral' hospitals, such as Mbagathi District Hospital and others soon reignited the suspicion that COVID-19 was a terrible illness with ill repute, much like HIV-AIDS a few years earlier.

The process of actually getting patients into those facilities took a while, and produced a most unintended poorly outcome: because the number of COVID-19 patients were few *and* entire major hospitals were isolated, the country ended up with the best hospitals lying idle as they awaited COVID-19 patients. It would be quite a long wait and was just as well. Most future non-COVID-19 patients would not, of free will, interact with any of the 'COVID-19-designated hospitals.' Communication on known COVID-19's transmission pathways and its possible lethality, but also on the government's actions to assure that all safety measures were being taken, was likely also influenced by the manner of dress by healthcare providers, who often appeared to be in 'space suits.' By implication, COVID-19 *had* to be especially severe or they would not need that kind of protection. Other implications are discussed elsewhere, but suffice to say, 'coronavirus stigma'[10] played a role in the excess deaths that were reported during the pandemic period.

Public Information and Communication: Institutions as Collaborators

Institutions (beliefs, tenets, rules) and organizations (civil, societal, and religious) are important in not only leading disaster response, but as partners in COVID-19 and especially in the case of COVID-19. The relationship between some religious faiths, congregations and traditions with vaccines and medical treatment has often imperiled the possibilities of containing and curing illness. While a discussion on 'vaccine hesitancy' in Kenya (more like vaccine unavailability) is considered in the next section, it is useful to highlight the role of communication and institutions in generating wider use and acceptance of measures that constrain religious practices but improve on the health of the nation. Of note, and perhaps rightfully contentious, is the limits imposed on religious practice on account of numbers.

Kenya's COVID-19 mitigation strategies have almost always included limits on religious meetings and congregations, eliciting quite the backlash from religious leaders. But a visit to any matatu stage, or to a supermarket, will show Kenyans tightly jam-packed in these facilities. Matatus flout social-distancing rules, and when you have 33+ people in a 33-seater Matatu, no argument can support the notion that social distancing is occurring. Further, some churches have exactly that many adherents and congregation sizes. Supermarket checkout lines are often equally crowded, as are the establishments themselves, with no limit on the number of shoppers who can be inside at any given moment. These contradictions strain government's credibility, especially when after reopening churches, political leaders use the pew as a perch for political purposes.

Organizations can be a positive force in the attempt to manage COVID-19. Most schools, for instance, complied with the directive to suspend activities until they were configured so as to minimize the risk of COVID-19. This affected even private schools, who depend on learners being present, in order to pay their employees, procure food (support the communities in their vicinity), among other things. By far the most closures stemmed from schools

---

[10] Alex Ayoyi, "*Low infection numbers fail to capture the impacts and stigma of COVID-19,*" *Africa at LSE* (22 Jul 2020). Blog Entry.

and universities. Religious institutions meet for far less time, potentially procuring less exposure, yet they were some of the most vocal entities about the need to reopen. Cooperation and coordination between such institutions and government is important, as was crafting strategies that did not punish one sector while allowing the functioning of the other, if the risk was almost equal. Institutions thus became half-hearted collaborators, but just as often sent out mixed signals given government's position on in-person meetings that its agents and even its own enforcers regularly flouted.

Public Information and Communications on Vaccines

The question of available information and public communication on COVID-19 vaccines has also split the nation, not necessarily because of a superior level of understanding of the science behind vaccines, but because of misinformation, disinformation, plain nefarious actors and even institutions dedicated to subversion of strategies they consider morally objectionable. While concerns about the speed of vaccine development (humans want slow, but also want a quick solution), there are rumors and hear-say that is unsupported by science, which public information could debunk. Kenya's problem with vaccines may revolve more around availability than skepticism, although both are highly prevalent, but the notion that some vaccines are made using derivatives of fetal tissue has been amplified by individuals, religious leaders and people of faith, casting doubt on their use and efficacy.

According to the US Centers for Disease Control and Prevention (CDC), "mRNA vaccines teach our cells how to make a protein – or even just a piece of a protein – that triggers an immune response inside our bodies"[11] without being infected with the virus itself. The process produces antibodies, so that in the event of exposure to the actual SARS-CoV-2 virus, the body already has generated antibodies that are then primed and ready to fight invading pathogens. In a 2018 article in the journal *Nature,* which had accumulated almost 2+ million views and published long before concepts such as mRNA entered every-day language, the science behind the mRNA technology was explicated, at the time attracting little to no attention. Then came COVID-19.

[11] CDC, "COVID-19: Understanding mRNA COVID-19 Vaccines," *The US Centers for Disease Control and Prevention*, Updated Mar. 4, 2021, https://www.cdc.gov/coronavirus/2019-ncov/vaccines/different-vaccines/mrna.html.

In the article, Pardi et al., highlighted some of the benefits of using newer technologies despite the many, initial difficulties encountered in doing so. The difficulties arose from a combination of insufficient previous research, the level of technological know-how and even the sophistication of the machinery used to create alternatives. Other limits included non-viability of *in vitro* mRNA transcription and the instability of the entire process. These challenges continued to favor the more traditional, "conventional vaccine approaches, such as live attenuated and inactivated pathogens and subunit vaccines [and] killed and DNA-based vaccines."[12] Yet with due respect to farmers, all, it is unlikely that Kinangop, Kitale, Kibwezi, or Kapsoet farmers are likely to become experts on the nuance of mRNA vaccines, the differences between them and the 'live attenuated,' and the impact, or not, on DNA.

This deficit provides an opportunity for government, one embedded in the duality of some level of dependence (and trust) in government, and prior dependence thereupon. Despite the clear, obvious and deep-seated historical, sometimes negative experiences with and at the hands of the government, it still *commands* the ability to coerce, to influence, if not to persuade. If and when public information disseminated in ways that alleviate the anxiety around vaccines generally, this would constitute a *proper,* non-propaganda, medical function of government. There is precedent: one rooted in Kenyans acceding to such vaccines as polio or BCG. Public information sessions, press conferences and currently non-existent health campaigns ought to address the misinformation, rumors, deceptions and related issues that fill the gap of a lack of information and that have been perpetuated by free access to crowd-sourced media platforms such as Facebook and WhatsApp. To wit, vaccines do not make people 'fat' on one side of the body, or make men impotent. Vaccines are not a European attempt at decreasing Africans' birth rate and its total population. They do not make people 'frigid' either. Nor is Bill Gates implanting microchips in people through the vaccine, and Africans are not being used as guinea-pigs for vaccine trials. These are some of the most salient, but by no means only rumors on COVID-19 in Kenya.

One might argue that especially in the era of liberalized media, sufficient information exists, so that citizens can make informed decisions on their own healthcare. But just as government regularly exercises legitimate use of force in enforcing rules including curfews it (and NERC) can provide good information to citizens. Disseminating centralized, credible, consistent and

[12] Norbert Pardi, Michael J. Hogan, Frederick W. Porter and Drew Weismann, "mRNA vaccines — a new era in vaccinology," *Nature Reviews Drug Discovery* vol. 17, (2018), 261 https://doi.org/10.1038/nrd.2017.243.

freely available information should be a default, an afterthought. Investing in resources to collect, analyze and dissemination so as to inform citizens is necessary. The Kenyan government already has such a model. It was first seen in the 1980s and 1990s with school broadcasts. Information broadcast should reach older Kenyans who are more vulnerable to COVID-19, are not on social media, and who might be persuaded to watch good information rather than Indian soap operas in local languages. NERC can and ought to have made it its business to explain the mRNA vaccines and communicate their safety: that they do not enter, or alter the DNA, and that vaccines are safe.

Public information campaigns are essential, especially given the rapidly-growing, well-established vaccine skepticism and hesitancy in Kenya but more broadly, especially across Africa, whose citizens interact regularly. For example, the 'Convince' compact (designed to encourage uptake of the - still scarce – vaccines, recorded one 'plugged-in' (to ICT) Nigerian (Moise) stating: "Our government is into fraud. They are saying there is coronavirus in Nigeria to make money."[13] Understanding these negative citizens' perceptions of African governments, including Kenya's, as 'into fraud,' including notions of 'COVID-19 Billionaires' is also understanding the distrust that governments have elicited, even over the question of COVID-19's existence. Neither are they helped by inability to account for foreign aid provided to combat the pandemic, or the perceived pumping of hundreds of millions of dollars into the sink-hole that is the World Bank's Kenya COVID-19 Health Emergency Response Project, which as of June 30th, 2021, had received US$246 million with nary a credible explanation as to the use of the funding.[14]

Perception of the COVID-19 vaccine being less safe than other vaccines is widespread.[15] The importance of eradicating the pandemic gives the government the responsibility of providing correct public information, and decreasing levels of distrust between citizens and science. A further source of the distrust arises from the negative historical experiences of citizens especially at the hands of the west (slavery and colonialism) and western vaccine makers, and the deficit of trust, honesty and sense of dependence that

---

[13] Rédaction Africanews, "Skepticism as COVID vaccination campaigns begin across Africa," *Africanews*, Last updated: 04/02/2021, https://www.africanews.com/2021/02/04/scepticism-as-covid-vaccination-campaigns-set-to-begin-across-africa.

[14] World Bank Group, "Kenya Secures $130 Million for COVID-19 Vaccines," *The World Bank Group*, Press Release, June 28, 2021, https://www.worldbank.org/en/news/press-release/2021/06/28/kenya-secures-130-million-for-covid-19-vaccines.

[15] Rumbi Chakamba, "Africans view COVID-19 vaccines as less safe than other vaccines," *DEVEX - Inside Development: COVID-19*, 25 March 2021, https://www.devex.com/news/africans-view-covid-19-vaccines-as-less-safe-than-other-vaccines-99451.

Africans might feel towards external vaccines. Yet, since we have lacked the capacity, know-how or leadership to develop our own vaccines, this creates the perfect damned-if-you-do, damned-if-you-don't situations. The website *Africanews* records Nigeria's experience with an experimental Pfizer vaccine in 1996 that resulted in 11 deaths,[16] yet government often insensitive policy of across-the-board, no-exemptions vaccination has often hurt, rather than helped build trust in vaccines.

Public information campaigns can also benefit from some of the most significant endorsements of science - those coming from sections of global religious leadership. For example, in the face of questions regarding the morality of the use of the vaccine, on 21 December 2020, the Vatican office with the charge of promoting and defending faith and morals, The Congregation for the Doctrine of the Faith expressed that "all vaccinations recognized as clinically safe and effective can be used in good conscience."[17] It clarified that such use of vaccines was neither cooperation with abortion, nor legitimating it: it was a moral responsibility to preserve life itself.

The statement also emphasized the voluntary nature of the vaccine, although it also cast vaccination in terms of the 'common good.' Hence, the statement articulated that, "*the morality of vaccination depends not only on the duty to protect one's own health, but also on the duty to pursue the common good*. In the absence of other means to stop or even prevent the epidemic, the common good may require vaccination, especially to protect the weakest and most exposed."[18] Such a powerful endorsement from the head of a 1.4 billion congregation is immensely powerful, and Kenya might do well to leverage it into public information campaigns available for public consumption, given the public waffling that the Kenyan churches were already showing.

The notion that the vaccine is somehow unsafe, religiously somewhat suspect or even insufficiently researched, absent medical evidence, in a country *simultaneously* immunizing against polio, is a target for government counter-programming. Indeed, educating the public about such vaccines as polio, which uses a more traditional form of live attenuated or inactivated virus

[16] Rédaction Africanews, "Skepticism as COVID vaccination campaigns begin," (2021), n.p.

[17] Laurel Wamsley, "Vatican OKs Receiving COVID-19 Vaccines, Even If Research Involved Fetal Tissue," *NPR – The Coronavirus Crisis – Coronavirus Updates*, December 21, 2020, https://www.npr.org/sections/coronavirus-live-updates/2020/12/21/948806643/vatican-oks-receiving-covid-19-vaccines-even-if-research-involved-fetal-tissue.

[18] Congregation for the Doctrine of the Faith, "Note on the morality of using some anti-Covid-19 vaccines," *The Vatican*, 21 December 2020, https://www.vatican.va/roman_curia/congregations/cfaith/documents/rc_con_cfaith_doc_20201221_nota-vaccini-anti covid_en.html.

as well as other viruses, or those who still use medical facilities, get medication and shots, trusting doctors and not knowing what is actually in the injections, is most interesting and countervailing. Kenyans have and will take other shots without questioning their doctors as to what the contents of the injection are but become quite knowledgeable when it comes to COVID-19 vaccines.

The public does have a solemn responsibility to obtain accurate information and avoid misinformation, but also perhaps extend some level of trust to the medical profession, the same one that they depend on for their other medical needs. After all, rarely do Kenyans ask to see a doctor's credentials before seeking treatment, or even most basically, ask to see a driver's driving license to ensure that they are qualified, before placing their lives in that vehicle. Whether or not the shots administered in public contain water or not, as some Kenyans might believe, is also an issue to be addressed, with confidence-building measures such as mass vaccination including of the public figures in ways that assure that the same batches of vaccine used on leaders are also the ones that are used on regular citizens, fighting misinformation to the contrary.

More broadly, a concise, well-coordinated, consistent and constant public information practice on all matters related to COVID-19, is critical to an informed, less skeptical and compliant public. But more than communication, compliance with the measures, whether by government or citizens, is critical as no amount of communication will help if the same government officials continue flouting the rules that they make, giving credence to the idea of *Wenye nchi* (the owners of the country) telling *wananchi* (citizens, or children of the country), what to do. It is also important to reassure the public that there are sufficient checks and balances to ensure that those visiting public health facilities for other reasons, such as seeking medical attention for other NTD among other illnesses, childbirth and overall medical wellness need to continue doing so. And most importantly, when they are available, vaccines' safety and efficacy will be important topics for public communication and information dissemination.

Institutional Disaster and Pandemic Management: Government by Committee? – NERC

Kenya has some history of disaster management, one that has been primarily associated with the military, police and fire-fighting brigades. However, the COVID-19 pandemic has necessarily required new planning 'infrastructure' to contain the pandemic. In review, The Kenya National Disaster Operation Center (NDOC) was established in 1998, after the 1997 El Niño floods that resulted in damage to crops and property worth over US$150 million.[19] NDOC's primary mandate was disaster preparedness, disaster management, relief coordination and overall reporting functions for disasters occurring in the country on a full-time, 24-hour basis. It was tested early, with the 1998 US Embassy bombing August 7th, and found to be rather ineffective as discussed in parliamentary proceedings recorded in the Hansard on February 5th, 2009.[20]

Noting the lack of preparation, an MP offered that: "I was a victim of a disaster in 1998, in the Co-Operative Bank. It took five hours for the Israeli Army rescuers to reach the site [...] the rescue team that had come all the way from Israel, five hours after the incident had taken place [...] who came and did the job that the Kenya Government was supposed to do?" NDOC did not feature much in public discourse after 1998; however, during the 2013 Westgate Mall Al-Shabaab terrorist attack, and was the first official government agency (body) to tweet on the attack, followed by local and international media houses as well as government agencies later on.[21] In principle, upon receiving reports of disasters, the NDOC would swing into action to ensure coordinated responses.

However, despite the NDOC's rather moribund existence, the pernicious, health-oriented nature of the coronavirus pandemic almost by default required a whole new approach to managing the public health disaster and emergency management, since it differs from a natural disaster. In a remarkable, anticipatory strategic move, the Ministry of Health crafted the 'National 2019 Novel Coronavirus Contingency (Readiness and Early Response) Plan' in February 2020, covering the February-April 2020 period, beginning the early stages of planning to combat the pandemic.[22] Some of the most pressing issues leading to the thinking on coordinating the COVID-19 response was Kenya's location as an international, even global and especially Africa's transit hub,

---

[19] Andre Yitambe, James Okello, C. M. Ooko Nguka, Caroline Ochieng and Ana Peña del Valle, "Road Traffic Accidents as an Everyday Hazard: Kisii and Kisumu, Kenya," In Mark Pelling and Ben Wisner, Eds., *Disaster Risk Reduction: Cases from Urban Africa*, (New York: Routledge, 2009).

[20] Kenya National Assembly, "Kenya National Assembly Official Record (Hansard)," 5 Feb 2009, (Nairobi: Government Printing Office, 2009).

[21] Suzi Migrani, "Spectacles of Terror: Media and the Cultural Production of Terrorism," In *Nele Lenze, Charlotte Schriwer and Zubaidah Abdul Jalil, Eds., Media* in the Middle East: Activism, Politics, and Culture, (New York: Palgrave Macmillan, 2018).

[22] ThinkWell Strategic Purchasing for Primary Health Care, "COVID-19 Summary Update for Kenya," (Washington, DC: ThinkWell, 2020). COVID- 19 Uganda updates (thinkwell.global).

"with 70% of international passengers being on transit,"[23] an issue of concern given the viruses then-unclear but suspected various transmission modes.

The National Emergency Response Committee (NERC) was the second major item of organizational and institutional planning. It came to life through the President's Executive Order No. 2/2020 on 28th February, 2020, days before the first COVID-19 case was diagnosed in Kenya. NERC was actually a combination and integration of the Cabinet's previous [[ad hoc]] Committee on Health and the Ministerial Technical Committee on Government Response to the Coronavirus, which were dissolved upon the establishment of NERC. Its membership comprised primarily of principals and their deputies in charge of different ministries and government agencies, and other administrators such as medical directors and liaison to the Office of the President; Cabinet Secretaries (CSs) and Principal Secretaries (PSs) in the ministries, supplanted by several offices and officials in charge of the public-facing services most prone to the vagaries and negative impacts of COVID-19.

NERC's precise membership included Cabinet Secretaries (CSs) for Foreign Affairs, Transport (and other portfolios), Development & Public Work, Defence, ICT (and other ministerial portfolios); Principal Secretaries for Health, National Treasury, Interior & Citizen Services, Transport, Telecommunications and Broadcasting, the Chair, Council of Governors (CoG) Health Committee; Directors (Immigration, Public Health and Medical Services - Kenya Defence Forces) and Directors General of Medical Services, the aviation regulatory body (Kenya Civil Aviation Authority) and the Kenya Airports Authority. The Office of the President's (OP) representation was by three officials: the Chief of Staff, the Principal Administrative Secretary and the Government Spokesperson. At its formation, NERC's designated chief officer was the Heath Cabinet Secretary, Mutahi Kagwe.[24]

NERC's mandate was self-evident, but involved taking the lead in "upscaling Kenya's level of preparedness and capacity to prevent, respond and contain [this] emerging global threat."[25] Other NERC tasks included coordinating the country's "preparedness, prevention and response to the threat of the Coronavirus Disease,"[26] capacity-building and coordinating medical

[23] Executive Office of the President (Kenya), "Executive Order No. 2 of 2020: National Emergency Response Committee on Coronavirus," The Executive Office of the President: State House – Registry, 28th February 2020, URL: https://www.health.go.ke/wp-content/uploads/2020/06/Executive-Order-No-2-of-2020_National-Emergency-Response-Committee-on-Coronavirus-28.2.20.pdf.

[24] Executive Office of the President (Kenya), "Executive Order No. 2 of 2020," (2020).

[25] Executive Office of the President (Kenya), "Executive Order No. 2 of 2020," (2020), 3.

[26] Executive Office of the President (Kenya), "Executive Order No. 2 of 2020," (2020).

personnel and other professionals for quick response and surveillance, including at all ports. Such surveillance was conducted on and directed at residents, citizens, crews and foreign nationals entering the country based on very limited entry criteria, particularly from COVID-19 hotspots, and determining quarantine needs and facilities.

Further, NERC developed, coordinated and largely implemented nation-wide and devolved-government level strategies, providing expertise to medical facilities, test kits, PPE, medications and therapeutics. It would also assess pandemic economic impacts and develop mitigation strategies such as developing human, technical and financial capacity internally and with partners and stakeholders, determining safe, effective and non-negative impact-resumption of business, travel and day-to-day activities. It was also mandated to, when necessary, co-opt individuals, groups and even institutions necessary to carry out its mandate.[27]

Although NERC's overall success at present cannot be conclusively determined, several of its members have become familiar faces at public briefings, some with a most impressive degree of humor (CS Mutahi), and some with concise medical information delivered as a doctor would (Dr. Mwangangi) and some with medical information infused with non-citizen-friendly, patriarch-minded, incomprehensible and outright rude explanations. NERC actively provides necessary information and updates, and its functions have been fairly well publicized. However, there has been a need to streamline communication about the structure of NERC, and coordination of the public information and briefing especially over activities of, and by the top leadership of the committee. It has especially been a necessary but overlooked reference to the guidance and directives being shown to be part of the NERC deliberations.

On the other hand, the notion that political considerations influence COVID-19 stats and numbers presented – once again, going back to the benefits of public information and of mis-communication, NERC's work and effectiveness is undercut by the impression that its decisions are driven by politics and that they aim(ed) to stymie one side of the political debate. For instance, rumors broadly suggest that, on a frequent basis, curfew extensions are informed not by the testing numbers (this is almost believable, given the extent of (non)-testing), but by political alignment. Since the government's Building Bridges Initiative (BBI) ran into judicial headwinds and Deputy President Ruto has continuously and actively held rallies, and has proven

[27] Executive Office of the President (Kenya), "Executive Order No. 2 of 2020," (2020).

increasingly popular over the outgoing president's preferred presidential candidate, the government generates numbers with high positivity rates to use as justification to impose curfews and limit in-person events simply to frustrate his political ambitions. It has felt suspiciously true.

Coincidence can especially be pernicious. After the July 2021 by-election in Kiambaa by-election, in which most reading of the election outcome was organic-egg-in-the-face for the ruling party's candidate, there is more interest in the government's COVID-19 'containment measures.' There is a corresponding but unrelated rise in the COVID-19 positivity rate, believed to be independently driven by the more contagious delta variant of COVID-19. The 'positivity rate' reached 13 percent on July 22nd, 2021.[28] The rising trend is not just in Kenya; rather, beginning with India, and now across the world, delta has shown itself to be mean and efficient. The coincidence might look like manufactured rage, but the jury is still out on that one.

Human Movement: Transmission+

Perhaps nothing is more impactful than human movement, or lack thereof. Movement is connected with life itself: health, work, nutrition, and nearly every other aspect of life. Cessation of movement, whether voluntary or not, has significant implications. When it is imposed by government, it may even border violation of basic human rights. But in the context of a global pandemic that was transmitted principally by humans, who are in close physical proximity or contact, generally within about three feet (or one meter)[29] of each other where one or more of the individuals is infected with the virus, symptomatically or even asymptomatically, *and* especially when aerosolized drops containing SARS-COV-2 virus are expelled into the air and subsequently ingested into the lungs, nose, mouth or eyes.[30]

---

[28] NTV, "COVID-19 Positivity Rate – 9:00 PM News Broadcast," *NTV,* July 22, 2021. https://www.nation.africa.

[29] While the WHO's FAQs suggest that 1 metre (about 3 feet) is the transmission distance of aerosolized droplets, CDC guidance and FAQs recommend 2 metres (about 6 feet). See: CDC, "COVID-19: Spread," COVID-19 Frequently Asked Questions, The Centers for Disease Control and Prevention, Page Last Updated May 25, 2021, https://www.cdc.gov/coronavirus/2019-ncov/faq.html#Spread.

[30] World Health Organization, "Coronavirus disease (COVID-19): How is it transmitted?" *Q & A – Coronavirus Disease (COVID-19)*, Updated 13 December 2020, https://www.who.int/news-room/q-a-detail/coronavirus-disease-covid-19-how-is-it-transmitted.

The asymptomatic transmission at close distances was the first issue for Kenya: considering that over 89 percent of urban travel is done using *Matatus*,[31] the frightening, undisciplined, overcrowded, personal-space-diminishing transport contraptions that ordinarily might be incubators of all manner of pathogens and their occupants harbingers of illness, if no measures were implemented, more than 90 percent of Kenyans might catch COVID-19 just by doing something ordinary and as simple as going to work, to the doctor's, or to undertake most daily activities. And because of the infrastructure, or lack thereof, the possibility of the now famous WFH – work from home – was almost non-existent. The most prudent, albeit painful decision then, might be to space out travelers in public transport, although that by itself would give rise to two new major issues: cost of transportation, and numericity.

The cost of transportation, especially in most Kenyan urban areas, and like most cities, whether one is considering HOV lanes or peak-off-peak travel, varies. In urban Kenya, it also varies with rain. Any slight disruption in 'normal' variation leads to even greater variation, but the transportation costs are both a result of bad planning (colonial policy and afterwards), the insanity of running just one commuter train in the morning and one in the evening to several of Nairobi's outskirts, and the start-end times for the normal business day. Despite the national 89 percent number of Matatu usage, in the three major cities, usage is estimated at 60 percent of families, 40-51 percent in 'midsized cities' and approximately 20 percent in other urban areas[32] (more commuters are more likely to use other public transport means such as motor-bikes, *boda boda* and others. In Nairobi alone, in 2009, the census showed a total of 3.1 million matatus in operation.[33] However, neither Nairobi nor more broadly Kenya, have solved the problem of public transportation, congestion or increased fares.

Planning transportation for the formal economy is vital, as is transportation for all manner of social, economic and individual activities.

---

[31] Deborah Salon and Sumila Gulyani, "Commuting in Urban Kenya: Unpacking Travel Demand in Large and Small Kenyan Cities," *Sustainability*, Vol. 11, No. 3823 (2019), 1-22 doi:10.3390/su11143823.

[32] Veronica Escamilla, Lisa Calhoun, Norbert Odero and Ilene S. Speizer, "Access to public transportation and health facilities offering long-acting reversible contraceptives among residents of formal and informal settlements in two cities in Kenya," *Reproductive Health*, Vol. 16, No. 1 (Nov. 8, 2019), 1-22, DOI: 10.1186/s12978-019-0828-0.

[33] Sarah Williams, Adam White, Peter Waiganjo, Daniel Orwa and Jacqueline Klopp, "The digital matatu project: Using cell phones to create an open source data for Nairobi's semi-formal bus system," *Journal of Transport Geography*, Vol. 49 (2015), 39-51 https://doi.org/10.1016/j.jtrangeo.2015.10.005.

Since they all depend highly on the semi-private public transportation network absent government capacity or competence to run an efficient transport sector, limiting commuting also impacts the organized economy and impacts the employment of those who work in the matatu sector. But more perniciously, it pits one of the most robust sections of the country's *id* against government, and against law enforcement, whenever that is the case, procuring rent—seeking opportunities for the law-keepers, defeating some public health measures and those very strategies the government purports to emplace in order to maintain public health.

Some of the calculations that citizens must do, even in the age of social-distancing, follow the classic Adam Smith's *self-interest,* in this case, getting to work. Because simultaneously COVID-19 did impact employment numbers and prospects, jobs are scarcer, and there is always someone else who might be willing to take risks, in addition to the lack of social support, getting to work *by any means necessary,* whether social distancing becomes a suggestion and the already scarce *Matatu* is flouting the guidelines, it is literally risk COVID or starve. It is also well known that most urban areas' and employers' formal day begins at 8 a.m., with few organizations exercising options such as flex time, even when customers patronize a business from 10:00 AM. Lunch is usually promptly at 12-1, while most organizations let out at 5 p.m. As such, there are concentrated crowds that emerge to put some pressure on public systems – transport and dining – like clockwork, early morning, lunch and 5 p.m.

Whereas this is not a discussion about integration of systems, like in many other sectors, the pandemic has laid bare the lack of planning, and the degree to which human activities depend on in-person interactions, without contingency planning for a 'perfect pandemic.' Besides the transport and formal work systems, work practices and even limitations have left head-scratching episodes, including the inability to work from home or whether COVID-19 transmits more after dark. Kenyan systems, similar to most African and surprisingly, even European countries, were not designed with proximate transmissibility pandemics in mind. Discussed elsewhere, it will be evident that other systems such as those educating the future in boarding schools, exam-based educational achievement systems, lack of basics such as internet and sporadic internet present no-choice choices, but also seek to upend those existing systems that took human contact as a given, even in such crowded places as matatus.

Constraining Human Movement: Curfews, Lockdowns and Travel Bans

In imposing the first curfew, which would later be followed a variety of movement restrictions – such as travel bans and lockdowns of counties around Nairobi as the COVID-19 case count climbed, the Kenyan Government was following what other countries across the world were doing *post haste* across the world. That said, Chukunzira casts Kenyan government's actions, in deciding to impose the curfew, in the following light: "the Kenyan state, as is, has inherited the colonial legacies of marginalization and exclusion and this has been highlighted in several ways in the midst of the pandemic."[34]

While it was announced only two days earlier, Kenya's first curfew was "imposed on 27th March 2020 from dusk to dawn to contain the spread of the virus. In practice, it means that from 7 p.m. to 5 a.m. all public spaces are off limits."[35] There were other unintended consequences that will later be highlighted as the full meaning and implementation of the curfew became a reality. These included access to income-generating means, and how the curfew would impact those who needed to work to eat, particularly without substantial, if any government assistance. The choice to starve or catch COVID-19, the partial title to another co-publication, was imminent.

The events of 27th March 2020, the first day of the daily, 7 p.m. to 5 a.m. curfew, not only illustrated the perfect storm of poor planning, but also of human rights violations, disregard for human life and on the whole, a worse outcome than actually dying from COVID-19. Two days previously, the president had directed, in his rather deceptively titled speech considering subsequent outcomes, item #15.1, "that effective Friday, 27th March, 2020; a Daily Curfew from 7 p.m. to 5 a.m. shall be in effect in the territory of the Republic of Kenya, with all movement by persons not authorized to do so or not being Medical Professionals, Health Workers, Critical and Essential Services Providers, being prohibited between those hours."[36]

---

[34] Angela Chukunzira, "Organising under curfew: perspectives from Kenya," *Interface: A journal for and about social movements*, Vol. 12, No. 1 (July 2020), 39 https://www.interfacejournal.net/wp-content/uploads/2020/07/Interface-12-1-Chukunzira.pdf.

[35] Chukunzira, "Organising under curfew," (2020), 39.

[36] PSCU, "Presidential Address on the State Interventions to Cushion Kenyans against Economic Effects of Covid-19 Pandemic," The Presidency – Briefing Room (Latest News), 25th March, 2020. https://www.president.go.ke/2020/03/25/presidential-address-on-the-state-interventions-to-cushion-kenyans-against-economic-effects-of-covid-19-pandemic-on-25th-march-2020/.

The crucial trouble arose in the curfew enforcement, which was provided for in the text of the president's directives of the same speech. Item #15.2 stated "that with immediate effect, the management of the Kenya Ferry Services is vested in the National Police Service, the Coast Guard and the National Government Administration Officers (NGAO)."[37] In this instance, NGAO (swahili, a word that can translate into 'shield') only served to protect the wanton violation of human rights that was captured on camera. In what is today acknowledged as the most problematic, criminal even, initial implementation of the curfew, the ferry was scheduled to shut down at 6:00 PM, but at 5 p.m., citizens were lined up – literally clobbered and whipped by overzealous 'law enforcement.'

The scenes shocked the nation, here and even outside the country, raising calls for the officers to be disciplined. Nonetheless, Kenya was not alone in this overzealous, rash, rushed, misunderstood and misdirected action to clear civilians out of the streets. Especially across Africa, these scenes were repeated severally. It would not be the only instance of government-sanctioned violence, carried out against civilians in the name of enforcing a curfew two hours before it was officially slated to start. The richest part of the irony was the killing of citizens long before COVID was even causing significant hospitalizations r even resulting in death. In Kenya itself, estimates of those killed by police during curfew enforcement range from 15[38] to 20[39] and recourse to justice is not assured.

Although curfews do limit the ability to move, the more restrictive travel ban and lock-down can have a significant, supplemental impact on constraining movement and therewith, the ability to provide for oneself. Maslow's hierarchy of needs would then dictate that individuals will likely consider what will kill them first: hunger might be more likely to do so considering the low rates of COVID-19-induced deaths, especially in Kenya. The economic sources of support, absent other social supports, had a similar effect on Kenya as did the lockdown in Italy's Lombardy region: people fled their abodes to places where they could either access food and housing with

---

[37] PSCU, "Presidential Address on the State Interventions," (2020), n.p.

[38] John-Allan Namu and Tess Riley, "Nine weeks of bloodshed: how brutal policing of Kenya's Covid curfew left 15 dead," *The Guardian/Global Development/Human Rights in Focus*, 23 Oct 2020, https://www.theguardian.com/global-development/2020/oct/23/brutal-policing-kenyas-covid-curfew-left-15-dead.

[39] Max Bearak and Rael Ombuor, "Police killed at least 20 Kenyans while enforcing coronavirus rules. Hopes for justice are fading," *The Washington Post*, 12/20/2020 https://www.washingtonpost.com/world/africa/coronavirus-kenya-police-shootings-curfew/2020/12/20/deb81d5a-3efc-11eb-b58b-1623f6267960_story.html.

little cost (up-country) or took refuge with relatives before the lockdown measures took effect. Since the number of infections in Kenya were still low to the extent that community spread was not occurring, it is unclear if such relocations contributed to any further infections.

The lack of social welfare support by government, prolonged curfews and lockdowns and overall economic downturns support Burlig's findings that short term lock-downs and temporary movement restrictions limit disease spread, but that long-term restrictions have the opposite effect, and are more likely to be flouted.[40] Besides restricting movement by its citizens within the country, Kenya's additional strategy to limit the spread of the virus included exclusion of foreigners other than those with 'valid residence permits' or returning citizens who would be required to quarantine in a 'government—designated quarantine facility,' another great source of controversy over both the cost and quality of facilities. Citizens who had entered the country over the previous fortnight were also required to self-quarantine.

The exclusion of foreigners and restrictions on most flights, other than those bearing cargo, into the country were slated to begin on 17th March, 2020. They would continue in one-month increments, or until as amended by the National Emergency Response Committee (NERC),[41] and by June 2020, there were facilities that allowed some residents and citizens to return. Occasionally, and in response to the fluid situation within the country, even domestic flights were limited for certain periods of time. For example, on March 29th 2021, with the rise in positivity rate and the imposition of stricter lockdowns and altered curfew hours, Kenya Airways and most other domestic carriers suspended all domestic passenger flights to Kisumu, Mombasa and other cities per new COVID-19 directives.[42]

---

[40] Fiona Burlig, *The Impact of Domestic Travel Bans on COVID-19 is Nonlinear in Their Duration,* (Washington, DC: NBER, 2021).

[41] PSCU, "Address to the Nation by H.E. Uhuru Kenyatta, C.G.H, President of the Republic of Kenya and Commander-in-Chief of the Defence Forces on Covid-19, Commonly Known as Coronavirus at Harambee House, Nairobi," The Briefing Room – the Presidency, 15th March 2020, https://www.president.go.ke/2020/03/15/address-to-the-nation-by-h-e-uhuru-kenyatta-c-g-h-president-of-the-republic-of-kenya-and-commander-in-chief-of-the-defence-forces-on-covid-19-commonly-known-as-coronavirus/.

[42] Elias Biryabarema, "Kenya Airways says suspends domestic flights after new COVID-19 lockdown announced," *Reuters, Middle East & Africa*, March 27, 2021, https://www.reuters.com/article/uk-health-coronavirus-kenya-airways-idUSKBN2BJ0CI.

COVID Curfews and Pandemic Inequality

The imposition of curfews, ban on movement and the shutting down of public facilities, including eateries and hotels, was the broader part of government actions to contain the pandemic. These facilities were required, in addition to observing the public health measures outlined by the health CS, to comply with other curfew and related COVID-19 measures articulated and designed to combat the pandemic; these included ending indoor dining services other than take-away food service. These imposed conditions produced a bit of creativity in way of response. Since eateries had an even more strict regime with earlier closing hours (mostly, around 4 p.m.), and the foods they could serve excluded most alcoholic beverages in a sitting, creativity included ordering sausages and beer or other similar combinations whose primary goal was less food and more drink.

Accordingly, "Kenyans would order a sausage or any other cheap foods in order to be served with drinks,"[43] in part to circumvent the government's largely despised attempts "to position itself as a father figure."[44] This was particularly the case due to the perception that the state (and especially the elites) was violating the rules itself, public officials were using the time and space to exact profit or revenge (including misappropriating donor-provided pandemic funding or demolishing buildings and individuals' houses and possessions). In the eye of the public, this the severity of the pandemic did not quite seem to be supported by the additional actions that were being witnessed.

Besides the question of allowing food establishments to serve alcoholic beverages, leading to the CS for Health announcing that citizens should not order 'one sausage and 10 beers' or whether bars and clubs were more likely to increase COVID-19 transmission than churches and the God-level implication of a 'praying nation' shutting down churches, and the KEMSA scandal that produced 'COVID-19 millionaires' overnight, the various iterations of curfews in Kenya since March 2020 have generated debate, but also great controversy. They have also been applied unevenly and in the parts of Kenya that are not Kenya (such as North-Eastern), even their application, and the challenge of pastoral communities and banditry can challenge the

---

[43] Knollyne Oindih Gai and Musa Nyakora, "Kenya's Leadership Response to Covid-19 Pandemic and Possible Interventions between March and June 2020," *East African Journal of Education and Social Sciences,* Vol. 1, No. 3 (December 2020), 113, DOI: https://doi.org/10.46606/eajess2020v01i03.0049.

[44] Gai and Nyakora, "Kenya's Leadership Response," (2020), 113.

effectiveness of curfews or the lockdowns, given the poor infrastructure and enforcement gaps.

Since March 2020, the texture, location, hours and strictures of curfew and its enforcement have varied with the rise and fall in the number of infections. Still, the country will have been under continuous forms and variations of a curfew, movement restrictions and lockdowns since March 27th, 2020. [45] For instance, as the curfew that was in effect in March 2021, a year after the first imposition, approached its scheduled sunset *and* at the same time, the positivity rate had climbed into the region of 22 percent.[46] Then, the Interior CS extended the 10 p.m. to 4 a.m. curfew by 60 days and the ban on public gatherings for another 30 days.[47] He also restricted the number of attendees allowed at any religious facilities for a further 90 days.[48]

Besides these renewed measures, 'COVID-19 hotspot zones' were identified, and additional measures crafted to contain the rising number of cases. This has especially been important given the rise and rapid spread of the delta variant, whose lethality and speed of spread is especially concerning. Kenyan research labs have successfully sequenced the SARS-CoV-2 genome and have a year's worth of experience,[49] but most testing facilities are not widely sequencing the genome despite the acknowledgment by Africa CDC, and WHO's recognition, that such sequencing is still the key to understanding and combatting the pandemic,[50] evidence from elsewhere shows the danger posed by new variants. For example, in the last week of June 2021 in the UK, the number of infections with the Delta variant increased from 33,630 to 75,953, which represented a 79% increase, and about 99% of all new cases

---

[45] PSCU, "Presidential Address on the State Interventions to Cushion Kenyans against Economic Effects of Covid-19 Pandemic," *The Presidency – Briefing Room (Latest News),* 25th March, 2020. https://www.president.go.ke/2020/03/25/presidential-address-on-the-state-interventions-to-cushion-kenyans-against-economic-effects-of-covid-19-pandemic-on-25th-march-2020/.

[46] Reuters Staff, "Kenya extends COVID-19 curfew by 60 days," *Reuters*, May 30, 2021, https://www.reuters.com/article/health-coronavirus-kenya-idUSL5N2NH072.

[47] Brian Ngugi, "Matiang'i extends night curfew by 60 days to curb Covid-19 spread," *Business Daily - Economy*, Monday May 31 2021, https://www.businessdailyafrica.com/bd/economy/matiang-i-extends-night-curfew-by-60-days--3419762.

[48] Huaxia, "Kenya extends curfew, ramp up vaccination to contain COVID-19," *Xinhua*, June 30th, 2021 http://www.xinhuanet.com/english/africa/2021-06/30/c_1310034770.htm.

[49] KEMRI / Wellcome Trust, "Kenya Scientists Release Genome sequencing for the Covid-19 Cases in Kenya," *Kenya Medical Research Institute (KEMRI) & Wellcome Trust*, June 1st, 2020, https://kemri-wellcome.org/zp-content/uploads/2020/06/Genome-sequencing-of-SARS-CoV-2-cases-in-Kenya.-Report-2-2.pdf.

[50] WHO, "Genome sequencing central to COVID-19 response," *WHO-Regional Office for Africa*, 25 February 2021, https://www.afro.who.int/news/genome-sequencing-central-covid-19-response.

identified as the delta variant even as the UK achieved and sustained probably the highest vaccination rate in Europe.[51]

The same variant, which begun to change Africa's fortunes in the aftermath of the devastation that it caused in India from March through June 2021, has been sequenced in Kenya, especially in the western region. This was part of the impetus that led to specific lockdown and curfew measures from June 29th, targeting 13 western counties, which were identified as new hotspots and were placed under an expanded curfew beginning 7 p.m. through 4 a.m. until July 31. The provisions also included limits on social activities such as burials and religious activities, and prohibition on public gatherings and any in-person meetings.[52] Ironically, and although correlation is not causation, suspicion abounds, that the Madaraka Day (internal self-rule) celebrations of 2021 which took place in Kisumu on June 1 may have had a hand in contributing to the rapid increase in the number of cases, particularly given the level to which public health measures were ignored including by the country's leadership.

Jirani and Complexity: Tanzania's COVID-19 Denials and Impacts

While curfews, bans on movement and surveillance on individuals entering the country is primarily a mobility-related issue that can be just as competently considered under epidemiological mitigation strategies, Kenya's bans on movement have been impacted by other external considerations. As a transit hub for most goods destined for the land-locked Great Lakes region, from the ports of Lamu and Mombasa, to the border crossings in Namanga, Busia and Nadapal among others, it is vital for trucks, especially, to transit through the country. That said, and given the very limited testing regimes that exist in most of the countries through which the road transit crews go through, Kenya's vulnerable responses to the COVID-19 pandemic was especially heightened.

The case of Tanzania's initial COVID-19 denials is especially pertinent. Tanzania's position is famously controversial, although the principal purveyor of these controversies was believed to have died of COVID-19 after a brief hospitalization in Kenya. Again, the value of transparent government

[51] Adrian O'Dowd, "Covid-19: Cases of delta variant rise by 79%, but rate of growth slows," *The British Medical Journal*, Vol. 373 (2021), doi: https://doi.org/10.1136/bmj.n1596.

[52] Gov.UK, "Foreign travel advice - Kenya," UK Government, https://www.gov.uk/foreign-travel-advice/kenya/coronavirus.

information-sharing cannot be over-emphasized. It would not do to suggest that after Magufuli's denials of COVID-19's existence, he then died of the same. Yet, with Africa believed to have "the world's greatest infectious disease burden [and] a weak epidemiological surveillance system," the COVID-19 denials did not just affect its citizens. As the 32nd largest country in the world and 13th in Africa, with a total of 4,161 land borders (with 1,424 km of coastline), of which 775km is shared with Kenya, this offered many opportunities for cross-border transmission of COVID-19, even with surveillance at Kenya's border crossings and OSBPs.

Tanzania's late president Magufuli famously expressed that the country's COVID-19 case counts and deaths were being inflated and were causing panic. He then promptly declared Tanzania COVID-19-free, stopped government efforts to track infections, and gave a most infamous televised national speech as to the reasons thereof. In it, he held that test samples that had included a goat, sheep, a paw paw, quails and oils were tested by the national laboratory, and returned false positives. That, he declared, was evidence that the testing was flawed, and that perhaps COVID-19 was not as much of a threat as it was purported to be.

Still, even with case counts continuing to climb in neighboring countries, there were not significant requirements for testing of Tanzanians entering Kenya, or denial of entry, as some governments had done with citizens of countries whose COVID-19 management and mitigation strategies were less than optimal. Indeed, while most – most – of the world was pledging to favor science over politics in managing COVID-19, Tanzania's Chief Medical Officer argued that "all we insist is that the research should be in line with national priorities,"[53] blind to the reality that COVID-19 has no respect for 'national priorities.' This is the classic case of individual decision-making which has sub-optimal outcomes for even other actors, particularly given that their shared border, peoples and economy provides for high levels of integration and interaction.

---

[53] Syriacus Buguzi, "Covid-19: Counting the cost of denial in Tanzania," *British Medical Journal* (Online), Vol. 373, (Apr 27, 2021). http://dx.doi.org/10.1136/bmj.n1052.

Chapter 2

Public Health Responses and Strategies: Basic Hygiene Responses

Abstract

This chapter examines the public health responses and strategies, focusing specifically on the basic health strategies and responses to the COVID-19 pandemic in Kenya. It begins by assessing the transmissibility of COVID-19, including a modest dive into the origins, classifications, mutations and variants that have been associated with COVID-19. The chapter details how SARS-CoV-2's anatomy makes it an almost perfect pathogen by increasing its transmissibility. It addresses some of the most basic mitigation strategies that might fall under the basic hygiene practices, including hand-washing and hand-sanitizing. In a nod to the proposed title (barakoa = mask), masks are discussed under the auspices of the Protective Personal Equipment (PPE). The anatomy of masks on Kenyan streets, including the 'peculiar' mask habits (chin-masks) and deleterious practices of sharing masks, is addressed. It addresses compliance with wearing masks, the habits of wearing and sharing masks, masks worn on the chin, and other peculiar practices. The responses and strategies included hand sanitizing, provision, cost and broad use of the Personal Protective Equipment (PPE) such as masks, lockdowns and mandates. The chapter especially focuses on and interrogates the practice of masks 'at half-mask' and masks at full mask upon the sight of police, reflecting on how public information on proper mask usage as a health concern rather than as a strategy to beat a fine or detention by police can change their adoption and proper use to combat COVID-19. It concludes that although masks have more benefits beyond the mere stoppage of COVID-19 transmission (especially in a country with air pollution as significant as Kenya's in urban areas), wearing masks can improve respiratory health while hand-washing and sanitizing can vastly improve overall basic health and combat the spread of other common hygiene-related diseases.

SARS-CoV-2: Anatomy of a Perfect Pathogen

The world has learnt, throughout the first approximately two years of the COVID-19 pandemic, that SARS-CoV-2 is a most pernicious, adaptive, persistent and deadly virus. It has come to appreciate (or has it), that as far as pathogens go, SARS-CoV-2 is almost *perfect.* Perfect, in a most destructive way. From its murky origins (thus concealing its source and the circumstances for its emergence) to the hypothesized pathway it took from animals (or lab) to other animals (humans), to its transmission pathways, even two years later, we are still in the grips of learning about it. Without endlessly rehashing the contentions about COVID-19's origins, there are those knowns, which have facilitated COVID-19's spread, and made the virus especially prone to transmission and the subsequent contagion, which was recorded as approaching 450 million cases and near 6 million deaths by the end of February, 2022.

For most people who find that their lives have been disrupted, indeed ended by COVID-19 – which is essentially everyone – the virus' subfamily (*Coronavirinae*) genomic signature, genetic and antigenic characteristics are likely fairly unimportant. But the impact itself is. The spike (S) protein might be of some importance, but the inability to breathe for those who are infected ad have to be placed on a mechanical ventilator, is especially frightening. The delta variant has been central to the more recent discussions, but that is driven more by its higher rate of transmissibility, up to 2.5 times higher than other variants, than by any other considerations as to what the spike protein or its mutation may look like. Even as the newer μ variant, which began to enter discussions in July and August of 2021, delta variant retained the highest transmissibility. But, the world would later come to learn of another even more 'efficient' variant, 'omicron', which though less deadly, was more contagious, thus doubling all previous records, including the total figure of 200 million (August 2021) to 450 million a short 6 months later.

Just as is the case with the families of coronaviruses, which until 2020 were the near sole domain of epidemiologists, it is useful to consider some of the COVID-19 attributes that make the virus so transmissible and eminently successful, even when some (significant) populations, including majorities, have been vaccinated. It is possible to do so without necessarily going deep into the SARS-CoV-~ weeds. SARS-CoV-2 is one of the 4 'genera' (α, β, γ, δ) coronaviruses that generally cause (severe) illness in humans, or those that are capable of infecting humans, and is specifically a β virus. It is related to other (genera of) coronaviruses that include SARS-CoV and MERS-CoV. Besides

SARS-CoV-2, other recent coronavirus illnesses and infections have included SARS-CoV, which is considered to transmit alongside (the more infectious, adaptive and transmissible) as well as SARS-CoV-2, Pangolin-CoV and Bat-CoV-RaTG13 viruses.[54]

Since its first appearance late in 2019, COVID-19 has been mutating rapidly, across strains, variants, states and populations, and seems to get 'better' with some of the variants and mutations. For example, as of February 2021, the US had recorded more than 670 mutations.[55] Across the world, the same was true, despite that discussing 'mutations,' 'types' and 'variants' can evoke confusion. Velázquez argued in April of 2021 that, "we know the coronavirus currently has 12,700 identified mutations, 12 main types of the virus (identified as 19 A, the original type, through 20 J), five strains and almost 4,000 variants."[56] The strains, adds Velázquez, "are known as L, […] the S strain followed by V and G (further mutating into GR, GH and GV, and several infrequent mutations collectively grouped together as O)."[57] Evoking even more confusion is the use of the Greek alphabet (alpha, beta, gamma, epsilon, and delta), which most individuals may not identify with and serves more scientific analytical purposes.

Formally, and as of the preparation date for this volume, COVID-19 has five major variants and thousands of mutations. The first was the 20A.EU1 or B.1.177 mutation,[58] which first appeared in Spain, the A222V B.1.1.7 (Alpha) variant was first seen in the UK, the B.1.351 (Beta) variant, first seen in South Africa, the P.1 (Gamma) variant, first detected in Brazil and the B.1.617.2 (or delta) variant, first detected in India and then rapidly becoming the most common variant across the world.[59] Two further variants were identified by

---

[54] Zhang Bao and Wei Zhao, "SARS-CoV-2: characteristics and current advances in research," *Virology Journal* vol. 17, No. 117 (2020), 1-17 DOI https://doi.org/10.1186/s12985-020-01369-z.

[55] William A. Haseltine, "What Are The 677 Mutations? New Covid-19 Variants Found In The US," *Forbes*, Feb 19, 2021, https://www.forbes.com/sites/williamhaseltine/2021/02/19/what-are-the-677-mutations-new-covid-19-variants-found-in-the-us/.

[56] Francisco R. Velázquez, "Coronavirus Mutations and Variants: What Does It Mean?" Spokane Regional Health District (SRHD), Apr 01, 2021, https://srhd.org/news/2021/coronavirus-mutations-and-variants-what-does-it-mean.

[57]. Velázquez, "Coronavirus Mutations and Variants," (2020), n.p.

[58] Sara Reardon, "The Most Worrying Mutations in Five Emerging Coronavirus Variants," *Scientific American - Public Health*, January 29, 2021, https://www.scientificamerican.com/article/the-most-worrying-mutations-in-five-emerging-coronavirus-variants/.

[59] CDC, "About Variants of the Virus that Causes COVID-19," National Center for Immunization and Respiratory Diseases (NCIRD), Division of Viral Diseases, The US Centers for Disease Control and Prevention, Updated June 28, 2021, https://www.cdc.gov/coronavirus/2019-ncov/variants/variant.html.

the Mayo Clinic; they are named Epsilon (B.1.427), and Epsilon (B.1.429).[60] It was established, based especially on UK data, that the delta (B.1.617.2) variant was 60% more transmissible than other variants, and was considered more dangerous.[61]

As of mid-July 2021, the delta variant was identified as the most rapidly-spreading variant, reversing the mitigation strategies adopted by different countries and that had proved to be fairly successful especially where and when vaccination numbers climbed, masks were more widely adopted, and the world settled into some sort of wait-and-see attitude. The most recent variant that appeared and extensively affected almost double the population affected by the previous four variants was Omicron, or B.1.1.529. As mentioned before, it was deemed to be less severe, but transmitted more easily, and thereby ended up sending more people to hospitals and needing care, given the sheer numbers involved. Even as Omicron ravaged vaccinated nations such as the US, as of January 24th 2022, BA.2 was classified as a newer Variant of Concern (VoC)+ based on the lineage of the Omicron variant.[62]

However, even as it mutates, epidemiologists have generally expressed the view that because SARS-CoV-2 is more stable than other viruses, including those associated with HIV, the mutations are less likely to change the basic structure of the virus, the care of those infected with the virus or the vaccines that are developed for the first mutations and variants notwithstanding the higher transmissibility, and thus, make it more likely that the virus can be combated successfully.63 Infectious disease experts have adjudged it to be changing more slowly – i.e., the different mutation sequences – are slower and less dramatic than, for example, the HIV virus.[64] That said, there has been some discussion over the efficacy of vaccines on the different variants, but the larger debate concerns whether COVID-19 will eventually become (or already has become) endemic after its pandemic status, thus

---

[60] Daniel C. DeSimone, "COVID-19 variants: What's the concern?" *Mayo Clinic – Health Information*, June 17, 2021, https://www.mayoclinic.org/diseases-conditions/coronavirus/expert-answers/covid-variant/faq-20505779.

[61] The Cleveland Clinic, "What to Know About the Latest COVID-19 Variant and Other Coronavirus Mutations," Cleveland Clinic – Health Essentials, June 22, 2021, https://health.clevelandclinic.org/what-does-it-mean-that-the-coronavirus-is-mutating/.

[62] WHO, "Tracking SARS-CoV-2 variants," The World Health Organization, February 2022, accessed on 2.26.2022 from: https://www.who.int/en/activities/tracking-SARS-CoV-2-variants/.

[63] Reardon, "The Most Worrying Mutations," (2021).

[64] Ewen Callaway, "The coronavirus is mutating — does it matter?" *Nature - News Feature*, 16 September 2020, https://www.nature.com/articles/d41586-020-02544-6.

requiring annual or at any rate, periodic shots that deal with the various variants.

The Structure of COVID-19's Transmissibility

When influenza-related pandemics have occurred, Kenya, and more broadly, Africa, has rarely been spared the deleterious effects of such pandemics though some have appeared to have less severe effects in Africa than elsewhere. Some of the impacts issue from the interconnected world in which we live, even back to the history of such pandemics as the 14th Century's devastating Bubonic Plague, the 20th Century Spanish Flu, or the 21st Century Ebola outbreaks. Respiratory-based pandemics are especially transmissible during these interactions. COVID-19's speed, transmission efficiency and infection rates have been compared to that of the Spanish Flu pandemic that ravaged the globe more than a century ago. And even in that pandemic, Africa, and specifically Kenya, had very dark outcomes, as the figures attest.

The Spanish Flu was highly lethal, with an estimated total death between 50 to 100 million of the 500 million people it infected, of a 1.5 billion population. About 33% of the world was infected; of these, 7% of those infected died. This compares to the 2.5% of the 7.6 billion (190 million) who have been infected by COVID-19 as of July 15th, 2021, with a death toll of 4.2, or 2.2% of those infected. The Spanish Flu was estimated to have a 20 percent mortality rate. Its lethality is attributed to a number of variables that include the respiratory and airborne transmission, its high rate of infection and simultaneously, efficiency; the poor levels of care, abysmal hygienic conditions, the almost comical (albeit repeated) mitigation strategies (lockdowns or parades) and the lack of a vaccine or cure. Wheelock reiterates that "the Spanish flu was highly contagious; it was also unusually lethal compared with a typical seasonal flu."[65] Unlike SARS-CoV-2's incubation period of anywhere from five days to weeks, H1N1 – the Spanish Flu – had a modest 1-2 day incubation period.[66]

---

[65] David Wheelock, "What Can We Learn from the Spanish Flu Pandemic of 1918-19 for COVID-19?" *Federal Reserve Bank of St. Louis*, Monday, June 1, 2020, https://www.stlouisfed.org/on-the-economy/2020/june/what-can-we-learn-from-the-spanish-flu-pandemic-of-1918-for-covid-19.

[66] Africa Center for Strategic Studies, "Lessons from the 1918-1919 Spanish Flu Pandemic in Africa," *Africa Center for Strategic Studies*, May 13, 2020, https://africacenter.org/spotlight/lessons-1918-1919-spanish-flu-africa/.

The broader geopolitical situation, i.e., the First World War and the mobility it provided, but the spread was helped along by the same war and the movement it brought, as the war came to an end. For the US, the estimated 45,000 deaths from the flu were only 8,000 less than those from the First World War.[67] Just as globalization, tourism and global supply chains have facilitated the spread of COVID-19, the-then global and colonial situation further facilitated the spread of the Spanish Flu. In Kenya, the Spanish Flu's impact was significant. The tally of an estimated 31,908 cases and 4,593 deaths associated with the Spanish flu in Kenya computed to 4 to 6 percent of the population, a number decidedly much lower than the British raj's close to 60 percent.[68] Kenya's trade with external and global markets, but especially the return of Carrier Corps who served in foreign armies during the First World War, "longshoremen and African soldiers returning from the European battlefields carried the disease into urban centers and their hinterlands."[69]

COVID-19's basic characteristics have not changed much from the very first patients in Hubei Province, although initially it was thought of as a 'flu.' These first patients reportedly "showed symptoms of viral pneumonia, including fever, cough and chest discomfort, and in severe cases dyspnea and bilateral lung infiltration."[70] These were the more severe symptoms; the milder symptoms generally "include fever, body ache, dry cough, fatigue, chills, headache, sore throat, loss of appetite, and loss of smell."[71] The latter became and especially important measure for possible COVID-19 infection, and conversely, became one of the ways individuals might test for the pathogen absent formal tests that were scarce, and continue to be so especially in Africa, with Kenya averaging less than 10,000 tests a day throughout the pandemic.

While we have collectively acquired much more knowledge on the virus over time, the images of patients being rushed to hospitals, getting intubated, doctors wearing 'space suits' to keep out the virus, browbeat doctors who couldn't help their patients and watched them lose the fight despite the growing hostility towards loss of freedoms and opposition to PPE and masks,

---

[67] Wheelock, "What Can We Learn?" (2020).

[68] Jürgen D. Müller, "Spanish Influenza in Kenya," Staff Seminar Paper No. 6 (1994/95), pp. 1 University of Hannover, https://www.academia.edu/31804192/Spanish_Influenza_in_Kenya.pdf.

[69] Müller, "Spanish Influenza in Kenya," (1994/5), 2.

[70] Ben Hu, Hua Guo, Peng Zhou and Zheng-Li Shi, "Characteristics of SARS-CoV-2 and COVID-19," *Nature Reviews Microbiology* Vol. 19, (2021), 141–154, https://doi.org/10.1038/s41579-020-00459-7.

[71] Harvard Medical School, "If you've been exposed to the coronavirus," *Harvard Health Publishing (Harvard Medical School),* June 02, 2021, https://www.health.harvard.edu/diseases-and-conditions/if-youve-been-exposed-to-the-coronavirus.

these heart-breaking 'struggles to breathe' were splashed on TVs across the world as the pandemic spread to Italy's Lombardy region and elsewhere. Here, Italy battled the pandemic in a most distressing fashion, which then spread to be replicated in nursing homes in Washington State and New York in the US, and most recently, the 'struggle to breath' and those ubiquitous huge oxygen tanks sought like gold and lugged to hospitals, and the accompanying desperation, spread to India.

The images haunted governments and doctors, citizens and scientists as patients and hospitals ran out of oxygen and families watched their loved ones gasping for the last breath that would not come. Within a few months, the whole world would be grappling with these same issues; some to a higher degree and some with more muted numbers. The virus's impact is enhanced by its airborne, aerosolized transmission It is believed to survive on surfaces for up to 24 hours, although the thinking behind this supposition has been increasingly challenged by new evidence, though at temperatures below 50°F (10°C), the virus' spread is much more likely. The World Health Organization (WHO) presents a more expanded list of modes of COVID-19 transmission, which include "contact, droplet, airborne, fomite, fecal-oral, blood-borne, mother-to-child, and animal-to-human transmission."[72] The spectrum of medium through which it can be transmitted vastly increases the likelihood of transmission, as it almost necessitates the complete end in physical interactions, particularly coupled with its longer, asymptomatic incubation period.

Typical of our fluid, changing but growing knowledge of COVID-19, current thinking suggests that its incubation period is ranges from a few days to even weeks. The duration of symptoms and incubation range from 2 days to 2 weeks, with an average incubation period of 5 days, 8 days for disease development, with intervening possible stays in the ICU, HDUs, comas and other intubated conditions generally following after this period. For most that succumb to the disease, death occurs within 16 days of initial (re) infection.[73] It also attacked those most vulnerable to the destructive power of the virus, perhaps predictably. Children have generally appeared less prone to the virus, and when they are infected, are generally asymptomatic. Additionally, "older

[72] WHO, "Transmission of SARS-CoV-2: implications for infection prevention precautions," *Scientific Brief*, 9 July 2020, https://www.who.int/news-room/commentaries/detail/transmission-of-sars-cov-2-implications-for-infection-prevention-precautions.

[73] Hu et al., "Characteristics of SARS-CoV-2," (2021).

people and/or people with co-morbidities are at higher risk of severe disease, respiratory failure and death."[74]

Other factors favoring COVID-19's seeming unstoppable spread is its 'high transmission efficiency' in a globalized 'international travel' regime.[75] Human social activities such as religious attendance have also been identified as potential 'super-spreader events,' where the COVID-19 virus is likely to utilize its unique capacities and suitable social and environmental conditions to spread unabated. For instance, a study in Brunei found that transmission was highest among spouses (~42%), through a religious gathering (~15%) and through children, by about the same margin, while household transmission was about ~11%, leaving 11% transmission unaccounted for.[76] That said, spouses likely live with children in households and attend the same religious services, in addition to the strategies that most governments utilized, such as lockdowns and bans on movement.

Basic Hygiene Responses and Mitigation Strategies

Hand Sanitizing

Even epidemiologists concede that the most important eradication strategy to deal with the COVID-19 pandemic is to stop its spread. As important as vaccines, therapeutics, use of PPE, sanitizing and social distancing are, elements of minimizing human contact between un/infected and can minimize the pandemic's spread even without all other mitigation strategies, particularly where universal vaccine availability is still light years away. But human beings are social creatures, and is evident, most of existing human systems – religion, education, work, politics – are all grounded on interpersonal human interactions. It therefore follows, that the first and often most effective COVID-19 mitigation strategies are based on limiting human contact, avoiding other humans especially those who might be infected, applying a cross-section of strategies to determine if one is infected (for example, use of 'infra-red thermometers'), and sanitizing hands and work-spaces to reduce

[74] Hu et al., "Characteristics of SARS-CoV-2," (2021).

[75] Hu et al., "Characteristics of SARS-CoV-2," (2021).

[76] Liling Chaw, Wee Chian Koh, Sirajul Adli Jamaludin, Lin Naing, Mohammad Fathi Alikhan, and Justin Wong, "Analysis of SARS-CoV-2 Transmission in Different Settings, Brunei," *Emerging Infectious Diseases*, Vol. 26, No. 11 (2020), 2598–2606. doi: 10.3201/eid2611.202263.

potential for transmission, and above all, wearing masks to contain droplets that might contain the COVID-19 virus.

The famous swahili saying, ‘heri nusu ya shari kuliko shari kamili’ (it is better half the trouble than the full complement of trouble) might apply to the practice of hand-washing, hand sanitizing and any other reference to the idea of using alcohol-based liquid compounds to kill the virus that might be transmitted through contact of any of the vector surfaces one comes into contact with. For the most part, hand sanitizing, generally abbreviated as 'sanitizing' in the Kenyan context, has become widespread, together with infra-red temperature checks using hand-held thermometers. It is not always clear what is in the sanitizing spray bottles, and one hopes that the contents are at least 70 percent alcohol content. They often look like water.

In the early days of the pandemic, and following Uhuru Kenyatta's call, public institutions, rather than private businesses, set up 'sanitizing stations,' which mostly entailed some water conveyance with faucets, and soap. The dearth of water often put a pin to the best intentions: proper hand sanitizing required a regular supply of soap, water and where widely used, alcohol-based hand sanitizers. At the same time, the World Bank and IMF were providing resources aimed at assisting the Kenyan government implement such necessary strategies as hand sanitizing, although it wasn't clear that the government, rather than private businesses, were best placed to do this especially given the subsequent 'COVID billionaires' saga that occurred after the money was disbursed. Thus, as important as hand sanitizing was, and has been, the fight for reduction of transmission was already imperiled.

Even before COVID-19, the importance of Water, Sanitation and Hygiene (WASH) had begun to attract the attention of donors, development organizations, increased advocacy from non-profits, and even philanthropic concerns such as the Bill and Melinda Gates Foundation. The logic thereof is clear: the general hygiene of most of the country's population, especially related to water-borne diseases, was abysmal. UNICEF had determined that "better water, sanitation, and hygiene could prevent the deaths of 297,000 children aged under five each year globally."[77] As COVID-19 made hand-washing that much more important, there were practical concerns, not only of lack of water, but also, of overcrowded informal settlements, sometimes referred to as 'slums.'

---

[77] UNICEF Kenya, "Water, Sanitation and Hygiene: Improving children’s access to water, sanitation and hygiene," *UNICEF – Kenya*, July 2021, https://www.unicef.org/kenya/water-sanitation-and-hygiene.

But even COVID-19 prompted creativity: for example, in the largest dumpsite in Kenya at Dandora, the UN housing agency, UN Habitat, together with other partners such as JICA and local residents, established a hand-washing station; a paradox, given that it is essentially a dump-site.[78] Even the young attempted to help; the story of a 10-year old boy who built a rudimentary hand sanitizing station tugged at the hearts of all and sundry, although his invention could not really be widely replicated or patented.[79]

Hand sanitizing can often seem perfunctory; it is done because the government directed business to make available hand-sanitizing stations, but the quality of the hand-sanitizers, especially inside spray-bottles, and the infra-red thermometers used in conjunction therewith, seem more useful in giving the impression that people are doing *something,* rather than that the 'something' being effective. With diluted hand sanitizers, some filled with decidedly suspicious concoctions, and with the process of sanitizing appearing to be more perfunctory to the extent that it complies with government directives more than being purposefully done to help contain COVID-19, the efficacy of sanitizing and hand-washing is suspect at best. On this, the ingenuity of Kenyans likely works against them.

Hand-sanitizing is only one of the mitigation strategies that are more visible than practical. One only needs to look at the lines of tightly packed-shoppers who congregate in super-markets, breathing down each other's' necks as they await to check out, to know that no amount of sanitizing, or queuing in the morning and especially evening, to catch *Matatus* home, without leaving the one-metre social-distancing gap, to understand the challenge that public health mitigation strategies face. One is well reminded of the old soviet saying, *they pretend to pay me, so I pretend to work.* Kenyans pretend to social-distance, hand-wash, sanitize and wear masks to the extent that it keeps them out of trouble with the authorities, not for its effectiveness.

[78] UN Habitat, "Hand washing stations in Nairobi's biggest dumpsite officially launched to tackle COVID-19 pandemic," *United Nations Human Settlements Programme – UN Habitat*, 9th March, 2021, https://unhabitat.org/hand-washing-stations-in-nairobi%E2%80%99s-biggest-dumpsite-officially-launched-to-tackle-covid-19-pandemic.

[79] Emily Moulin, "Nine-Year-Old Kenyan Boy Builds Hand Sanitizing Station To Help Fight COVID-19," *Dogonews.com,* August 10, 2020, https://www.dogonews.com/2020/8/10/nine-year-old-kenyan-boy-builds-hand-sanitizing-station-to-help-fight-covid-19.

Personal Protective Equipment (PPE), Masks and Mandates

Among the new COVID-19 vocabulary items that entered our consciousness was Personal Protective Equipment, PPE. Long before COVID-19 became *the* thing that disrupted lives, PPE was discussed in different settings and using the various terminology derived from such institutions as the International Standards Organization (ISO), NATO, US Title 29 (Code of Federal Regulations), the American Society of Testing Materials, the Japanese Institute of Standards (JIS) and other organizations and industries,[80] including Kenya's own Kenya Bureau of Standards (KEBS). The referent contexts include, for example, in chemical, biological and radiological work and potential situations.[81]

Some of the PPE that made widespread appearance in medical and care settings was already common, including during the Ebola crisis; others were less common. Later, one of the most globally ubiquitous signs of the COVID-19 pandemic was, is the proliferation of face masks. Indeed, one surmises that they are so widespread even the oceans depths are now finding that new pollutants include the different variants of masks. Other PPE is less easily disposed of, but it is clear that masks have become an important part of combating the pandemic since its early days.

Much has been written about Kenya's situation, especially with regard to COVID-19 and the impact of PPE, such as the pollution that manifested at the coast within the first 100 days of the mitigation strategies being implemented,[82] or more epidemiological observations such as the (sometimes otherwise impactful) reduction in amount of physical contact among the citizenry[83] due to selected mitigation strategies. What is perhaps less widely

---

[80] Eva F. Gudgin Dickson, *Personal Protective Equipment for Chemical, Biological, and Radiological Hazards: Design, Evaluation and Selection,* (Hoboken, NJ: John Wiley & Sons, Inc., 2019), n.p.

[81] Dickson, *Personal Protective Equipment,* (2019).

[82] Eric Okuku, Linet Kiteresi, Gilbert Owato, Kenneth Otieno, Catherine Mwalugha, Mary Mbuche, Brenda Gwada, Annette Nelson, Purity Chepkemboi, Quinter Achieng, Veronica Wanjeri, Joey Ndwiga, Lilian Mulupi and Jill Omire, "The impacts of COVID-19 pandemic on marine litter pollution along the Kenyan Coast: A synthesis after 100 days following the first reported case in Kenya," *Marine Pollution Bulletin*, Vol. 162, (2021), https://doi.org/10.1016/j.marpolbul.2020.111840.

[83] Matthew Quaife, Kevin van Zandvoort, Amy Gimma, Kashvi Shah, Nicky McCreesh, Kiesha Prem, Edwine Barasa, Daniel Mwanga, Beth Kangwana, Jessie Pinchoff, CMMID COVID-19 Working Group, W. John Edmunds, Christopher I. Jarvis and Karen Austrian, "The impact of COVID-19 control measures on social contacts and transmission in Kenyan informal settlements," *BMC Medicine*, Vol. 18, No. 316 (2020). https://doi.org/10.1186/s12916-020-01779-4.

addressed, are the attitudes amongst the citizenry towards the masks and/or face coverings, their attitudes towards enforcement of mask mandates, and the clash of ideas: between the COVID-19 skeptics and government enforcement of mandates, but also, the every-day small victories that citizens score through near-compliance, but with masks riding the chin, thus defying the government to perhaps do something about it, alongside giving support to the destitute and providing more social support given the pandemic's impacts.

Masks on Kenyan Streets

A sojourn into the streets of the major cities is like a journey into a country of thousands of (mis~) and different 'understandings' about COVID-19, the role of masks in combating the pandemic, their (in~) effectiveness and how to wear them. They come in all shapes, sizes, durability, consistency and styles. A most caustic ways in which they have been described was, 'kufungwa mdomo kama mbuzi' (being 'muzzled' like a goat) – or looking more like one of those race horses on Kentucky Derby day. A masked person does evoke the image of a Llama whose mouth is covered with cloth to stop them spitting. For the Kenyan situation, mostly 'medical grade' masks are used, although their consistency suggests that they are less than what one might find in other mask markets in other countries.

Although the Kenyan government, alongside the guidance provided by the WHO, the US CDC and Africa CDC, have been at the forefront of disseminating information on face coverings such as masks, cloth face coverings, gaiters and related 'aerosolized droplets inhibitors,' such guidance, and the masks themselves, are sometimes insufficient, inaccessible, unaffordable and the guidance unenforceable. Basic guidance includes cleaning hands before, after wearing a mask and after touching it, coverage of nose, mouth, chin, proper storage, washing and/or disposal (trash bins, medical waste), avoiding masks with valves and decidedly not sharing masks.[84]

The US CDC adds other important guidance such as widespread masking, social-distancing *and* wearing a snugly-fitting mask, full-time, use of masks in public gatherings as well as indoors even in spaces that are well—

[84] WHO, "Coronavirus disease – (COVID-19) advice for the public: When and how to use masks," 1st December, 2020, *World Health Organization*: https://www.who.int/emergencies/diseases/novel-coronavirus-2019/advice-for-public/when-and-how-to-use-masks.

ventilated, the age at which most persons in public should be spotting a mask (above 2 years), need for masking if living with someone in home recovery or care for COVID-19, removing masks from back to front without touching the mask, washing hands for at least two minutes after mask removal, but also, the liberty to not wear masks if one is alone or away from others or with members of their household with whom one usually lives with.[85] It further recommends the types of masks that should be worn: medical procedure masks (especially K-95), other surgical and medical procedure masks, breathable-materials masks (cotton), fabric mask (tightly woven fabric), as well as those not to wear: poor-fitting, leather or plastic masks, loose masks that let light through, one-layer masks and masks with nozzles and exhalation valves as well as scarf/ski masks.[86]

By themselves, other types of face coverings, such as face shields or neck gaiters are not recommended by the CDC, and in the age of Omicron, have been found to be merely decorative: they do not stop the transmission of the COVID-19 virus. Findings from a study by Lindsey et al. provide some insight and explanation as to why, even though Lindsey was not addressing the now newer Omicron variant. "An N95 respirator blocked 99% [...] (SD) 0.3%) of the cough aerosol, a medical grade procedure mask blocked 59% (SD 6.9%), a 3-ply cotton cloth face mask blocked 51% (SD 7.7%), and a polyester neck gaiter blocked 47% (SD 7.5%) as a single layer and 60% (SD 7.2%) when folded into a double layer. In contrast, the face shield blocked 2% (SD 15.3%) of the cough aerosol."[87] Although the efficacy of the medical, K-95 masks and their equivalents is considered to be higher, these were often reserved for the medical workers and were mostly unavailable in countries such as Kenya.

That said, K-95 or N95 (medical-grade) masks offered better protection than other masks, although even surgical and medical masks had significant efficacy. For example, "the filtration efficiencies of various cloth masks and a medical procedure mask, it was estimated that the better fit achieved by combining these two mask types, specifically a cloth mask over a medical

---

[85] CDC.Gov, "Guidance for Unvaccinated People – Guidance for Wearing Masks," *US Centers for Disease Control and Prevention*, Updated Apr. 19, 2021, https://www.cdc.gov/coronavirus/2019-ncov/prevent-getting-sick/cloth-face-cover-guidance.html.

[86] CDC.Gov, "Guidance for Unvaccinated People – Guidance for Wearing Masks," (2021).

[87] William G. Lindsley, Francoise M. Blachere, Brandon F. Law, Donald H. Beezhold and John D. Noti, "Efficacy of face masks, neck gaiters and face shields for reducing the expulsion of simulated cough-generated aerosols," Aerosol *Science and Technology*, vol. 55, No. 4 (2021), 449-457, https://doi.org/10.1080/02786826.2020.1862409.

procedure mask, could reduce a wearer's exposure by >90%."[88] Further research and better understanding of the different layers of, and materials used to make the masks, has led to a decreased on the near prescription of N95 masks use. Research has shown near parity in the levels of protection that various masks offer. For instance, facing insufficient supplies of medical, and sometimes surgical masks, various establishments have resorted to recycling, sterilizing and otherwise refreshing masks, or recommending the use of cloth masks when the recommended types are unavailable. But one cannot say the same for the medical grade masks that are reused again and again, only being subjected to washing. In most settings, such masks are discarded after three to four hours.

The question then is one of the levels of protection that these non-original masks provide has been a key determinant as to the guidance that has been available. However, research found that "expired N95 masks and sterilized N95 masks provided the same level of protection as new N95 masks with greater than 95 percent filtration."[89] There was a marked decrease with other masks similarly treated: "surgical masks with ties provided 71.5 percent filtration, while surgical masks with ear loops only provided 38.1 percent."[90] More recent CDC guidance has demonstrated that "multi-layer cloth masks can both block up to 50-70% of these fine droplets and particles, and limit the forward spread of those that are not captured."[91] It is worth repeating that even as variants emerge, some will defy the expectations and violate the known tenets; we keep learning.

Research also showed that double-masking was marginally more effective, albeit by paltry 1-2% improvement over the use of a single surgical mask.[92] It is useful to consider the context of this guidance and its application

---

[88] John T. Brooks, Donald H. Beezhold, John D. Noti, Jayme P. Coyle, Raymond C. Derk, Francoise M. Blachere, and William G. Lindsley, "Maximizing Fit for Cloth and Medical Procedure Masks to Improve Performance and Reduce SARS-CoV-2 Transmission and Exposure, 2021," *CDC - Morbidity and Mortality Weekly Report (MMMW)* No. 70 (2021), 254–257. DOI: http://dx.doi.org/10.15585/mmwr.mm7007e1.

[89] John T. Brooks and Jay C. Butler, "Effectiveness of Mask Wearing to Control Community Spread of SARS-CoV-2," *JAMA Insights*, Vol. 325, No. 10, (February 10, 2021): 998-999. doi:10.1001/jama.2021.1505.

[90] Brooks and Butler, "Effectiveness of Mask Wearing," (2021), n.p.

[91] CDC, "Science Brief: Community Use of Cloth Masks to Control the Spread of SARS-CoV-2," *The US Centers for Disease Control and Prevention (CDC)*, Updated May 7, 2021, https://www.cdc.gov/coronavirus/2019-ncov/science/science-briefs/masking-science-sars-cov2.html.

[92] Emily E. Sickbert-Bennett, James M. Samet, Steven E. Prince, Hao Chen, Kirby L. Zeman, Haiyan Tong and William D. Bennett, "Fitted Filtration Efficiency of Double Masking

to Kenya. Though Kenya's pandemic surveillance, detection, containment and treatment capabilities continue to grow, much guidance on mitigation strategies has generally mirrored that of the major scientific and medical organizations' such as CDC, WHO, Africa CDC, KEMRI and others and practices seen in the developed countries, with some local modifications, e.g., social distancing at between 1, 1.5 and 2 metres as opposed to CDC and most international health organizations' consistent standard of 6 feet (2 meters), one trusts that the virus behaves the same way in most environments and therefore, the guidance even on social-distancing should be consistent.

Kenyans' 'Peculiar' Mask Habits

Whereas 600 days is arguably a long time to wear masks especially in public and under potential sanction of fine and arrest, Kenyans have somewhat adapted to the practice. Like everywhere else, these masks have seen certain modifications and beautification, but also creativity in what passes as a mask and quite as often, incorrect practices of wearing masks. The Kenyan government has not been as effective at communicating some of the numbers and the impact of the proper wearing of masks, even though the level of skepticism over whether even COVID-19 itself exists drives the practices witnessed. Before examining some of these, it is also useful to note that unlike the guidance in other areas of the world. Elsewhere, particularly where government provides masks, use of other face-nose-mouth coverings, such as bandannas, gaiters and scarves is less prevalent than in Kenya. The question is often one of whether it is better to have a weak form of 'masks', such as the bandannas, or whether they create a false sense of security. That said, asking people to buy masks to protect against something that they are not quite convinced is a threat to them, as most Kenyans perceive COVID-19, leads to high levels of creativity.

This was especially the case in the absence of that debate, and the immediate shortage of KN95/FFFP devices.[93] Indeed, lack of viable

During the COVID-19 Pandemic," *JAMA Internal Medicine - Research Letter,* (April 16, 2021), doi:10.1001/jamainternmed.2021.2033.

[93] Jeremy Howard, Austin Huang, Zhiyuan Li, Zeynep Tufekci, Vladimir Zdimal, Helene-Mari van der Westhuizen, Arne von Delft, Amy Price, Lex Fridman, Lei-Han Tang, Viola Tang, Gregory L. Watson, Christina E. Bax, Reshama Shaikh, Frederik Questier, Danny Hernandez, Larry F. Chu, Christina M. Ramirez and Anne W. Rimoin, "An evidence review of face masks against COVID-19," *Proceedings of the National Academy of Sciences (PNAS)*, Vol. 118, No. 4 (Jan 2021) e2014564118; DOI: 10.1073/pnas.2014564118.

alternatives to the recommended surgical masks served to feed into the suspicion that some government bureaucrat was benefitting from importing the different COVID-19 management and mitigation supplies such as masks. At the same time, Kenya ought to have been well-placed to pivot to the making of cloth-based face coverings. In 2017, it banned the use of plastic bags, with hefty fines promised, of up to Kshs. 4 million (or 4 years' imprisonment) for manufacturing, importing or selling plastic bags.[94]

Most of the plastic bags manufacturers retooled to produce cloth-based bags, which often have the texture and consistency of face masks, albeit perhaps not as significant protection against viruses. It is likely that there was further retooling of the same to produce dyed, near-medical masks which have now proliferated the market. To assist with the production of medical-grade and re-usable masks, the International Finance Corporation (IFC) helped Kenya's Hela Clothing makers retool their clothes' production and shift to making masks, which have been distributed across the East and Central African region. This is useful, considering the production challenges and supply-line delays that have affected practically all of the resources used to fight COVID-19, as the major global manufacturers saw increasing infections and implemented their own mitigation strategies, decreasing global trade.[95]

Some creativity in masks does exist, although most masks are the 'standard' surgical masks, of different colors. Organizations too, have often produced, or commissioned masks – perhaps as a way of keeping their employees safe, but equally, as a way of advertising. However, there has been less color and creativity in this area, perhaps illustrating the conservative nature of Kenyan society and peoples. Simultaneously, more entrepreneurial citizens have taken to creating masks, some of which look suspiciously cut out from cloth and other materials such as coarse garments. These solve some of the old-age *angst* produced by masks, especially the 'chafing effect' behind the ear. Still, most of the available masks remain the single-use, 3-hour-limit surgical mask. One dare not even venture into the reality of single-use masks worn over several days, not hours.

---

[94] Republic of Kenya, "The Environmental Management and Co-Ordination Act," *The Kenya Gazette - Special Issue*, Gazette Notice No. 2334, Vol. CXIX, No. 31 (14th March, 2017), https://www.nema.go.ke/images/Docs/Awarness%20Materials/Gazette_legal_Notice_on_carrier_bags.pdf.

[95] Mary-Jean Moyo and Tania Lozansky, "Working with Africa's apparel makers to produce personal protective equipment," *Nasikiliza (World Bank Blogs),* May 19, 2020, https://blogs.worldbank.org/nasikiliza/working-africas-apparel-makers-produce-personal-protective-equipment.

Deleterious: The Practice of Sharing Masks

Given the government-imposed requirement that masks be worn in most public settings by most but the youngest and medically (respiratorily) vulnerable, and the levying of 'instant' fines on offenders, to the tune of Kshs. 500-1,000 per person per offense, citizens who forgot to being masks with them, or did not want to wear them or for one reason or another, and did not have alternative face coverings, found themselves scrambling to either buy masks at Kshs. 10 per piece, or borrow from 'well-wishers.' Whereas this has often been the very last resort, individuals have in the past been known, recorded even, as borrowing sometimes pre-used masks. Certainly, living in multi-person households where any hope of social distancing, especially in the slums, and re-using pre-used masks is likely to result in a higher probability of infection, and spread of the pandemic, *in spite of* masking.

The challenge of 'sharing' masks is not only present in Kenya; it has also been recorded in countries like Nigeria, where research found "unhygienic and ill-advised use and sharing of masks especially multiple fittings before buying from vendors." There are other factors associated with higher probability of sharing masks. For example, people who (bum) share cigarettes are more likely to share masks; thus, "sharing a cigarette was associated with higher risk of [COVID-19] infection."[96] But government policy often drives the inevitable poor choices that citizens make. Overall personal and country economic conditions are also significant in the choices that citizens make: indigent persons who might otherwise want to conform to government policy might consider the economic consequences and choose food over purchasing masks, figuring the latter might kill one slowly.

With regard to government policy, in March 2020, anyone found not wearing masks, flouting existing social distancing, or not following hand-sanitizing rules was subject to a fine of Kshs. 20,000, be imprisoned for 6 months, or both.[97] In a country where this, as a fine, constitutes over 10% of the average annual per capita income, and might entail significant loss of freedom, borrowing masks becomes a matter of course, since one might just

---

[96] Pawinee Doung-ngern, et al. "Associations between Wearing Masks, Washing Hands, and Social Distancing Practices, and Risk of COVID-19 Infection in Public: A Cohort-Based Case-Control Study in Thailand (6/18/2020)," http://dx.doi.org/10.2139/ssrn.3633162.

[97] Citizen Reporter, "If you fail to wear a mask in public, you risk Ksh.20,000 fine or 6-month jail term," *Citizen Digital*, April 10, 2020, https://citizentv.co.ke/news/if-you-fail-to-wear-a-mask-in-public-you-risk-ksh-20000-fine-or-six-month-jail-term-329499/.

as easily die in jail as from COVID-19. An early report from the informal settlements in Kibera demonstrates the effects of the government's mandate:

> To avoid being on the wrong side of the law, a section of needy Kenyans are now sharing masks. Some borrow from their neighbours when they have to go to public places. In some residential places, one face mask is shared among ten people. This is very dangerous since the disease can easily be transmitted from one person to another.[98]

Indeed, if there was a case of 'the road to hell' being paved with good intentions, government policy that causes citizens to share masks in order to avoid arrest and imprisonment at a time when only 8 COVID-19 deaths had been recorded, this ought to make the list.

Masks at Half-Mask

A most curious practice has receded in recent months, occasioned by a crackdown by police officers on masks worn to cover everything except COVID-19's transmission pathways. This has been the persistent practice of wearing the mask under the chin, so that the mask only covers the chin, essentially leaving uncovered the most significant transmission pathways, i.e., the mouth and nose. Because the initial requirement was to 'wear a mask' as opposed to 'correctly wear a mask,' the practice of masks under the chin, hence *'Barakoa for my chin,'* became widespread. The irony was that technically, citizens 'had' and were 'wearing' masks, but were doing so improperly. In fairness, if the government had not specified how they should be worn, then it was inevitable that they would be worn haphazardly, and given their constraining effect on breathing, one understands why *chin masks* were *in*. But on the other hand, it magnified citizens' lack of appreciation of the objectives of masks, to stop COVID-19, but a broader skepticism towards the whole enterprise.

Combining the various challenges associated with masks in Kenya - perceived high cost, at between Kshs. 10 and 50 per piece (and hence un/affordability), use, borrowing, sharing and especially failing to use them properly, a health representative in Kibera in Kenya noted that: "many people

[98] Samuel Ouma, "COVID-19: Are Destitute Kenyans Sharing Masks?" *Pan African Visions*, April 14, 2020, https://panafricanvisions.com/2020/04/covid-19are-destitute-kenyans-sharing-masks/.

have the masks but they use them inappropriately. Some keep them in their pocket while others are hanging them on their necks, *others covering the chin* while others are holding them in their hands. I think they only have them because it is now illegal not to have masks in public places,"[99] [my emphasis] illustrates the ambivalence of the public to take COVID-19 seriously, observe public health measures, or to properly use the masks outside of the threat imposed by possible financial penalties or being jailed.

There has been a marked improvement in the wearing of masks by Kenyans, even though it is not clear that the protection is even approaching the paltry 38 percent protection for masks worn with just ear-loops and without other modifications that improved the efficacy of masks. But equally, an unhealthy number of Kenyans will regularly pull down their mask when having a conversation, and leave it at chin level. This not only defeats the purpose of wearing the mask in the first place, because by pulling it down and expelling (and simultaneously possibly inhaling) aerosolized droplets, this is the moment of greatest vulnerability to infection. Further, the masks are generally of lower quality, fit less snugly, and wearing them on the chin has them completely removed from any orifice that produces or ingests the aerosols. To this extent, masks are worn not for the protection that they provide, but to avoid fines and penalties if and when one should be stopped by the police.

Masks at Full Mask: The Sight of Police

As noted earlier, pandemic mitigation strategies have been vigorously enforced by the national government through the use of police officers, often with such zeal that enforcement resulted in death. Kenyans are often victims of aggressive policing, but more significantly, the zealous enforcement of COVID-19 rules is less about containing the pandemic than about potential rent-seeking opportunities and just plain harassment of citizens. Besides the catch-22 situation, where not having a mask leads to a possible arrest and placement in overcrowded, unhygienic cells that are likely better disease vectors than say, walking along a street in the open, without a mask, and without clear guidance on whether (although one presumes this to be the case)

---

[99] Peter Mwangi Kibe, Lyagamula Kisia, and Pauline Bakibinga, "COVID-19 and community healthcare: perspectives from Nairobi's informal settlements," *Pan African Medical Journal*, Vol. 35 (2020), 1-3, (Suppl 2): 106. doi: 10.11604/pamj.supp.2020.35.24532.

the arrested are provided with masks or they might pick up new infections, the cash-bail and quarantine conditions provide incentive to attempt to get out of those circumstances.

Both parties – the individual and the police officer - have an incentive to conclude the matter quickly, and lucratively, at least for one side, while the other side essentially decreases their potential cost. In an interview conducted in the early days of the pandemic in Kibera, respondents suggested that "it is cheaper to bribe the police than go for the compulsory quarantine if found outside during the curfew hours or not wearing a mask" and blatant admission that bribery is cheaper, faster and more efficient than the justice system, even though it is unclear what it does to the public health issues. "When you are arrested without a face mask or after 7 P.M., you bribe your way out quickly. You call your mother or friend to give money to the police for your freedom. If you are taken to quarantine what will your children eat?"[100]

On the question of wearing of masks, the government was more forceful (and threatening), avoiding the dilly-dallying seen in other countries such as the US, where the guidance on masks continued to evolve and to be contested. Whereas in countries like the US, wearing of masks was impacted by many considerations, such as notions of 'liberty,' or perceptions that "culturally, the U.S. wasn't really prepared to wear masks,"[101] masks were similarly alien to Kenyans. But the threat of being arrested and being forced to quarantine of violators was effective, primarily because the enforcers, the police, have established a record of enforcing rules (existing or not) with a zeal, and not paying up (a bribe) is often seen as a point of personal victory by citizenry. Still, there was going to be that little measure of victory: it would be worn, but around the chin.

Occasionally, the enforcement efforts run afoul of the citizenry. For instance, in mid-2020, a policeman was beaten up by citizens from the Kibokoni area in Mombasa, with the citizens alleging that the police officer was harassing them (to wear masks). He ended up in hospital. A police station was burned in Kisii on July 6th, by residents who were protesting the killing

---

[100] Patrick Mutahi, Kate Jane Wanjiru, "Police Brutality and Solidarity during the COVID-19 Pandemic in Mathare," 2020, https://mambo.hypotheses.org/2895. ffhalshs-03078529.

[101] Nina Bai, "Still Confused About Masks? Here's the Science Behind How Face Masks Prevent Coronavirus," *Patient Care – University of California San Francisco*, June 26, 2020 https://www.ucsf.edu/news/2020/06/417906/still-confused-about-masks-heres-science-behind-how-face-masks-prevent.

of a trader merchandising masks and sanitizer.[102] A report in April 2020 by Transparency International (TI) reached similar conclusions: that enforcement of COVID-19 measures in Kenya created a pathway for police officers to seek avenues for personal enrichment through bribe-taking. It is clear then, that even though citizens are careful to avoid getting in trouble over not following COVID-19 rules, zealous enforcement of COVID-19 mitigation strategies can and produced unintended consequences, and continue giving the virus space to spread.

Although a discussion on the implications of COVID-19 on societal corruption is addressed in a different section of this piece, it is worth noting that besides Transparency International, the World Bank and IMF and other IFIs that have been instrumental in availing funding to help Kenya combat the pandemic, and calling out the COVID-19 billionaires, single-sourcing of medical equipment and no-bid procurement processes, even locally, there is recognition that COVID-19 has provided opportunities for petty corruption. When the Inspector General (IG) of the police forces is prompted to suggest to the public, that, "do not offer or give any bribes to anyone," there is both an inelegant admission of the existence of the practice and its widespread nature in the age of COVID-19, but also implicitly, that his men, women and non-binary persons are often less than credible partners in the fight against COVID-19. Such are the implications of a pandemic running rife through a bandit nation.

Public Information on Masks

To increase effective use of masks by the public, there is need to highlight the benefits of the proper use of masks. For instance, the government would do well to publicize the findings reported by the US EPA on the efficacy of masks and other PPE as they were tested in EPA's labs in Chapel Hill, NC. The government and ministry of health ought to communicate more clearly to the public, that the 71.5% protection (filtration) is achieved with surgical masks with ties, 38.1% by masks with ear loops only, a 3-layer knit-mask provided 26.5% of particles similar to aerosolized COVID-19 particles, 2-layer woven nylon masks with filter provided 79% protection, while tightening ear loops

---

[102] Andrew Kasuku, "Tables turn: Mob beats up cop after confrontation over a mask," The Star, 11 July 2020, https://www.the-star.co.ke/news/2020-07-11-mob-beats-up-cop-after-confrontation-over-a-mask/.

on commonly used medical masks, securing masks with rubber bands and even using the much-hated brown stocking over a mask increased protection by almost 20% to 80 percent.[103]

Communicating other benefits of masking, especially in a country where clouds of dust are as numerous as the citizens themselves ought to be part of government strategy. Not only are masks quite effective, when properly worn, in stopping the transmission of COVID-19; they also have other health and medical benefits, such as filtering dust and other particles out of the air we breathe. Further, as the government continues to build new – especially road – infrastructure, the benefits of wearing masks can only increase. Whereas it is the case that masks can make breathing difficult, one ought to carry out a cost-benefit analysis, and the benefit will mostly come out on top. Still, there is need for other common-sense practices: family members riding in a private motor-vehicle ought not to need a mask, unless they have to also wear one in their private residential settings.

The Last Word on Masks

Hindsight is generally said to be 20-20: we often see things more clearly long after they are not immediately urgent or relevant. As much as wearing masks might annoy the general public, hide our faces and even potentially impede speech development because kids cannot adequately pick up on non-verbal cues, masks can have secondary, beneficial health effects. History has shown the widespread use of masks especially in China and Japan even where there was no pandemic or other respiratory outbreaks. Masks can be beneficial in places and environments with higher air pollution (China makes this list), where there might be higher probabilities of catching other pathogens (for example, the annual influenza virus) or dirt. Kenya is especially well represented in this last category as the amount of dust and fumes swirling in the air is to be marveled at.

Besides masks, the benefits of other recommended and widely practised health and hygiene practices in the age of COVID-19 are worth considering for the long term. Hand sanitizing, social distancing and avoidance of handshakes sound like really good hygiene practices. Most joke that one never

[103] EPA, "EPA Researchers Test Effectiveness of Face Masks, Disinfection Methods Against COVID-19," United States Environmental Protection Agency, Published April 5, 2021, https://www.epa.gov/sciencematters/epa-researchers-test-effectiveness-face-masks-disinfection-methods-against-covid-19.

knows where another's hands have been, and it does not hurt to wash and now, sanitize them before eating, greeting and doing other activities that require their use. It is almost the case that COVID-19 has uncovered our deeply (sometimes) unhygienic practices, and showed us that we have been quite minimalist with our hygiene practices, and beyond the pandemic period, we would be well-served by adopting these practices long-term.

Chapter 3

Public Health Strategies: Epidemiological Responses

Abstract

This chapter examines public health's more advanced epidemiological responses to the COVID-19 pandemic in Kenya. It examines one of the most controversial elements of COVID-19 management in Kenya: the use of quarantine and quarantine facilities. It discusses the quarantines and facilities, highlighting their often sub-standard and prohibitively costly facilities, leading to those placed in quarantine fleeing confinement and creating peril for other citizens. Testing, tracking and tracing, considered to be a critical part of the toolkit for dealing with the pandemic, is largely absent in Kenya, which brings into question the whole strategy of epidemiological responses. The chapter addresses the dearth in testing in Kenya (there have been 5X more vaccine doses administered as of February 2022 than there have been tests done), and the contravening evidence from seroprevalence. The chapter also addresses those infernal vaccines and their challenges (stigma, unavailability, suspicion of containing harmful substances) and the broader, more global controversies such as the proposition of Bill Gates tracking people somehow using the vaccines. The chapter also addresses government strategies and pronouncements regarding vaccine-for-access – to critical government services, and the implication thereof, considering the (un)availability of the vaccines. The chapter addresses broader issues with consistency of government policies with realities on the ground, and the need for government to continue sensitizing individuals and the public as to the benefits of the vaccines in returning back to a 'normal' life.

Quarantines and Quarantine Facilities

Separating those who are ill with potentially contagious pathogens has been a well-worn strategy. Even as far back as the era of the Black Death (the Bubonic Plague) in the 14th Century, those who caught the plague were abandoned to their fate. Those who were clear of the Bubonic Plague often formed communities, essentially isolating themselves to ensure they would not catch the plague. This may have been one of the earliest recorded elements of quarantine. For parts of Europe, these communities in quarantines eventually began the Italian Renaissance period. During the 1918 Spanish flu, related practices of quarantine were also witnessed. As such, quarantines are neither new, nor unexpected in the management of a pandemic. The changes that have used more recently target those infected or exposed to the COVID-19 pandemic, rather than the broader public. Kenya has had some experience with the latter, although this related to the stigmatized patients who were diagnosed with the HIV-AIDS virus particularly in its early stages.

The first instances of quarantine in the era of COVID-19 in Kenya did not go well. In fact, they went terribly wrong, as was recorded by Human Rights Watch (HRW). Whereas HRW is often accused of engaging in hyperbole as it seeks to highlight human rights abuses (at least, if you as African governments), the screaming 'headline,' 'Kenya Stops Abusive Forced Quarantine Related to CoVID-19,' might have produced a chuckle, were it not an accurate reflection of what the government had been doing up to that moment.[104] Besides the poorly condition of the quarantine facilities, the treatment of those entering quarantine by both medical officials and everyone else who was helping man the facilities discouraged anyone entering the quarantine facilities. Public attitudes did not help either; the level of stigma that COVID-19 attracted made it almost impossible that one could contract COVID-19 and have it treated as just another respiratory illness.

Although Facebook is not a reliable, academic or quotable source, it is an interesting and useful space to understand public opinion on certain issues. For example, public debate relating to COVID-19 and whose part commentary was posted to NTV Kenya's Facebook post included a religious leader (Reverend) quoted thus: "The bible speaks of quarantine for those who had leprosy."[105] Additional commentary includes; "Leprosy was quarantined because [sic] was transmittable like so corona."[106] Therein, one can see both the public perception of the pandemic (equated with, compared to leprosy) and

---

[104] Tenzin Wangmo, "Kenya Stops Abusive Forced Quarantine Related to Covid-19: Officials Launch Guidelines for Self-Isolation of Covid-19 Patients," *Human Rights Watch*, July 31, 2020 https://www.hrw.org/news/2020/07/31/kenya-stops-abusive-forced-quarantine-related-covid-19.

[105] NTV, *NTV Kenya Facebook,* (Web), Persistent ink: http://ow.ly.kiZP50yQTIj available at: https://m.facebook.com/NTVKenya/photos/a.80240814057/10156405017714058/?type=3 &locale2=zh_CN.

[106] NTV Kenya, *NTV Kenya Facebook*, (2020).

the religious angle that conflated leprosy with coronavirus, even though other more transmissible diseases such as Ebola, Marburg Fever, or even HIV-AIDS have not seen that level of religious fervor of separation of those infected. One needs not restate the consequences of attaching stigma to an illness – these have been especially deliberated in the case of India and COVID-19.[107]

Quarantine constituted another of the Kenyan government's strategies outlined in the initial planning steps in March 2020. According to Kenya's Ministry of Health, "quarantine is separation and restricted movement of well persons presumed exposed often at home or may be in designated residential facility or hospital. It can be applied at the individual, family or community level."[108] The initial quarantine areas were to be in the designated facilities until sufficient community spread had occurred; then, it would move to occur in more residential settings. It was not quite clear how this, with the known overcrowding, the multiple-generation single home occupancy and overall crowding in the said homes would work without increasing the infection rates and numbers.

NERC's plan called for the establishment of government-run 'quarantine' facilities. Because now movement was limited, this implied that there were those who had already entered the country within the previous 14 days, the widely-acknowledged virus incubation period. Therefore, it was medically justifiable and necessary to separate recent entrants from the public, so as to minimize the chances of transmission, particularly given the-then mediocre testing regimen. But just as the case with almost everything around the pandemic resembled barely-managed chaos, implementation of the quarantine, selection and cost of facilities oscillated between comical and tragic, leading to the suicide of a South African national who had found herself in quarantine, in the earliest days of the pandemic. There was a reported world of wrong about the facilities, some of which is explored next.

---

[107] Vaishnavi Chandrashekhar, "From leprosy to COVID-19, how stigma makes it harder to fight epidemics," *American Association for the Advancement of Science - Science* Sep. 16, 2020, https://www.sciencemag.org/news/2020/09/leprosy-covid-19-how-stigma-makes-it-harder-fight-epidemics.

[108] Patrick Amoth, "Interim Guidelines on Management of COVID-19 in Kenya: COVID-19, Infection Prevention and Control (IPC) and Case Management," *Ministry of Health*, https://kma.co.ke/Documents/Case%20management%20protocol.pdf.

The Quarantine from Hell

In hindsight, the quarantine practice and philosophy were in keeping in line with (a mind-boggling) practice found widely in some Kenyan institutions and practices. Citizens are regularly detained in hospitals and medical facilities – especially maternity wings – until they settle any outstanding (medical) bills, thereby accumulating even *more* charges. One surmises that this is a self-defeating strategy because, if one is unable to pay a smaller bill, how would one afford to pay a bigger bill *especially* if they are confined and unable to pay the smaller bill. COVID-19 saw a repeat of this, with the individuals who were initially sent(enced) to these facilities. That 200 persons in quarantine escaped from the KMTC facility in Nairobi was both tragic but almost understandable; "these people don't understand why they are in quarantine, they see it as punishment [...] in the government facility [that] the government should take care of you because if you tell someone from Kibera to pay 2,000 shillings a day. This person earns 10,000 a month. How is he going to pay for that?"[109] Granted, 50 of the escapees being subsequently arrested drinking did not exactly help their cause.

The cost of self-quarantine made it inevitable that anyone. finding themselves in any facility would do their best to *not* be there longer than a few short minutes, and there were frequent 'help' signs held up for journalists, evoking hostage situations. The facilities selected ranged from hotels to university dormitories, and other aesthetically less-appealing places attracted steep costs: a princely US$100 a day, about US$1,400 – US$1,700 for the two-week COVID-19 virus incubation period, without accounting for food costs, other necessities but also aggravations. Although this was on the higher side, there were other tales of horror; for instance, a returnee from Dubai, UAE, was to be quarantined for 14 days, but spent 32 days at a cost of US$434, which was (interestingly) negotiated down to US$$65. The individual finally departed the facility after being "often cold, hungry and so frightened that she said she blocked the door at night with an empty bed."[110]

For citizens, this amounted to almost their entire yearly earnings as measured by GDP per capita, *and* in the absence of any stated government

---

[109] Mohammed Yusuf, "COVID-19 Pandemic: Kenyans Confined at Quarantine Facilities See It as Sentence," *VOA News,* April 22, 2020, https://www.voanews.com/covid-19-pandemic/kenyans-confined-quarantine-facilities-see-it-sentence.

[110] Abdi Latif Dahir, "Kenyans Held for Weeks in Quarantine Were Told to Pay to Get Out," *The New York Times – Africa*, May 8, 2020, https://www.nytimes.com/2020/05/08/world/africa/kenya-coronavirus-quarantine.html.

social intervention strategies and food/rental assistance, quarantine would be a hole no one would ever dig out of. Even residents, nationals and citizens, and crews arriving in Kenya from abroad, the notion of traveling 10,000+ or more (or less) miles, just to be stuck a few miles from home, was not helpful. Having to be at a quarantine facility became a most distressing proposition, so distressing that the BBC termed it as being "sentenced" to a quarantine center. One can see why: "the toilets are just messy, dirty… even the cleaners who clean the toilets once a day complain how messy the toilets [...] It's because there is no water, so people are touching the same taps when you want to wash your hands, if there is even water… it's just a mess."[111]

Even more unhelpfully, as HRW pointed out, quarantine conditions were facilitating, rather than reducing transmission by "forcefully quarantining tens of thousands of people in facilities that lack proper sanitation, protective equipment and food."[112] Additionally, those tasked with managing the quarantines "have also held crowds of people in the arrivals area at the Nairobi airport for more than four hours with no social distancing, sanitizers, or masks; ferried people in packed buses with little ventilation; and, at the quarantine facilities, failed to enforce quarantine guidelines issued by the Health Ministry."[113] The very objective of enforcing social-distancing thus becomes most problematic.

Police officers were regularly accused of sending pregnant women to quarantine facilities contrary to Ministry of Health and NERC guidance. At the same time, there was denial of access to hospital for expectant women. Considering the potential peril that expectant women might face, given that vaccines were not initially authorized for expectant women, was utterly unconscionable – not to mention the obvious denial of human rights. Transportation of individuals rounded up and destined for quarantine facilities imperiled the police officers themselves and potentially, their families. The NGAO officers regularly used overcrowded transport trucks with poor ventilation, crammed together with the violators; this exposed them to potential infection, and subsequently, their own families.[114]

---

[111] Basillioh Mutahi, "Coronavirus: The fear of being sentenced to a Kenyan quarantine centre," *BBC News*, Nairobi, 20 April 2020, https://www.bbc.com/news/world-africa-52326316.

[112] HRW, "Kenya: Quarantine Conditions Undermine Rights: Ensure Access to Health Care, Sanitation, Information," *Human Rights Watch,* May 28, 2020, https://www.hrw.org/news/2020/05/28/kenya-quarantine-conditions-undermine-rights.

[113] HRW, "Kenya: Quarantine Conditions," (2020), n.p.

[114] Frank Ojwang', "Human Rights Violations During COVID-19 Curfew in Kenya: When Poverty Increases Chances of Preventable Death," In Stefan Kirchner, Ed., *Governing the Crisis: Law, Human Rights and COVID-19*, (Zürich: LIT Verlag, 2021).

An interesting question is on which individuals get hit with quarantine orders. The crowded streets of Nairobi – and other major cities – inspire no confidence that excluding foreigners from entry, or requiring them to go to into quarantine and to subsequently emerge into the crowded, no-mask, no-social-distancing, sketchy-sanitizing protocols reality that is Kenya, is as practically self-defeating as it sounds. Kenyans exhibit lackadaisical attitudes towards COVID-19. The government insists on self-isolation, quarantine and other related measures even as it requires negative PCR tests or evidence of having recovered from COVID-19 as a condition for entry by any new arrivals, without exemption for vaccinated foreigners, residents and citizens, as source countries ramp up vaccinations. The reality of political leaders who flout COVID-19 rules and do not have to quarantine undermines government efforts at enforcing its own rules, evoking a sense of *wenye nchi* against *wananchi.*

There are other more devastating outcomes of quarantine, especially during the first days of its implementation. The suicide (by hanging) death of a South African woman who had been placed in a 14-day mandated quarantine at the Kenya Industrial Training Institute (KITI) in Nakuru in March 2020, after complaints of poor conditions at the facility was tragic, even unnecessary. But more than the tragedy, and whatever other underlying conditions, it was a most poignant indicator that better planning and placement was necessary, and placing individuals into such inhospitable conditions, with some complaining of lack of basic needs, and services was going to procure bad outcomes. Facilities that the government selected for quarantine, together with the requirement to pay for sub-standard facilities was an affront. Rationality ought to dictate that people would consent to quarantine if the government took responsibility over quarantine costs payment *as a public health necessity.*[115]

The need to protect public health, even at cost, ought to be of higher concern than charging individuals the cost to quarantine. Even as COVID-19 passed the 500th day and the new, rapidly-spreading delta and newer variants continue to overwhelm nations, it is important to learn from the many mistakes that the government, the ministry of health and the police forces have made, and continue to make, as they implement public health directives. This includes the police's own well-being but also, ensuring that quarantine is not so flawed as to actually spread the virus, rather than contain it, as intended.

---

[115] Kiprotich Kimetto, "South African woman quarantined in Nakuru commits suicide," *Citizen Digital*, March 27, 2020, https://citizentv.co.ke/news/south-african-woman-quarantined-in-nakuru-commits-suicide-328133/.

ABCs of COVID-19 Management: Testing, Tracking and Tracing

One of the areas in which the Kenyan government has consistently failed – with a possible F-grade – is in testing. As of July 15th, 2021, the Ministry of Health update indicated that a total of 2,036,472 total tests had been performed, representing 3.81% of Kenya's total population tested. This also computes to 4,072+ tests per day.[116] In comparison with the US, 476 million tests had been reported as of July 12, 2021 (some sources show more than 490 million). This computes to a staggering 144% of the US population tested,[117] a figure that illuminates the gap between the possibilities of testing outcomes, even with the challenges that many African countries, Kenya included, have experienced with access to testing kits, antigens, capacity, know-how and related matters.

Troublingly, when testing has occurred, Kenya's positivity rate has oscillated between a low of about 4%, a middling rate of about 18% in November 2020 and a high of 22% in March 2021. OCHA Data further supports this notion that Kenya is not testing enough; for example, Kenya reached 1.04 million tests on December 30th, 2020, while the US on the same day hit 255.6 million tests, about 77% of its computed population, with almost 3 million tests performed on that day alone in the US.[118] Granted, other aspects of US COVID-19 management were catastrophic, but testing, track and trace and low-cost mitigation strategies have been highlighted as central to pandemic management. From the very beginning, there were calls for mass-testing, particularly in informal settlements where the living conditions were more likely to support community spread.[119]

Testing, tracking and tracing in Africa, whose numbers lag those of other regions by significant numbers, is not because of a lack of knowhow; rather, a combination of policy, infrastructure, skeptical citizens and the combined effects, help account for some of these outcomes. For example, "by March 7,

---

[116] Ministry of Health, COVID-19 Update, 15th July 2021, *Ministry of Health, Republic of Kenya*, https://www.health.go.ke/.

[117] CDC, "COVID Data Tracker," *Centers for Disease Control & Prevention,* Updated July 15th, 2021 from: https://covid.cdc.gov/covid-data-tracker/#cases_totaltests.

[118] OCHA Services, "Total COVID-19 Tests Performed by Country," *Humanitarian Data Exchange* (HDX), 15 July 2021, https://data.humdata.org/dataset/total-covid-19-tests-performed-by-country.

[119] Rachel W. Mbogo and John W. Odhiambo, "COVID-19 outbreak, social distancing and mass testing in Kenya-insights from a mathematical model," *Afrika Matematika* (2021), https://doi.org/10.1007/s13370-020-00859-1.

2020, laboratories in 43 African countries could already do COVID-19 testing."[120] Africa's progress here has been surprising, given that it "leads much of the world in community health-care networks that could be mobilised for the hard work of communication, testing, and contact tracing"[121] especially given its experience with Ebola and other highly contagious diseases. It has also shown the capacity to test for contagious diseases such as HIV, with a number of countries conducting millions of HIV tests within 3 months (Oct 1 – Dec 31, 2019 - South Africa conducted 7.3 million).

Testing for and detecting a new virus required the rapid development of new tests. With the approval of a new Polymerase Chain Reaction (PCR) test and other antigen tests, most of which were developed and manufactured for the developing world, saw Africa suffer from (new) COVID-19 Test Nationalism: just as developed countries have purchased and hoarded many millions of vaccine vials, even those not approved for use in their care systems, most of the developed countries want to test and test and re-test their citizens to the 140% rate, while African countries remain unable to test beyond the low single digit percentages of their entire population. This led to the UN concluding that even with the assistance of governments or individuals such as Jack Ma and his donation of COVID-19 tests, "the continent falls very short from the tens of millions tests the UN estimates will be required."[122]

That said, Africa's reported 3.4 million COVID-19 tests performed by June 2020 (1,700 tests-per-million), were celebrated as progress "on a continent starved of economic and health resources."[123] One might consider these though, to be self-inflicted wounds. Africa has never especially focused on self-reliance in the healthcare sector to the extent that it should have developed integrated research infrastructure capable of producing COVID-19 tests without relying on the Global North. And even the ability to develop its own tests early on did not solve the problem of scaling up production of test kits and more recently, of COVID-19 vaccines despite loosening up of IPRs and patents. Today, many African countries' COVID-19 strategies and reactions continue to be funded by the more prosperous countries of the Global

---

[120] Matthew M Kavanagh, Ngozi A Erondu, Prof Oyewale Tomori, Victor J Dzau, Emelda A Okiro, Allan Maleche, Ifeyinwa C Aniebo, Umunya Rugege, Charles B Holmes and Lawrence O Gostin, "Access to lifesaving medical resources for African countries: COVID-19 testing and response, ethics, and politics," *Viewpoint*| Vol. 395, No. 10238 (May 30, 2020), P1736 DOI: https://doi.org/10.1016/S0140-6736(20)31093-X.

[121] Kavanagh, et al., "Access to lifesaving medical resources," (2020), 1736.

[122] Kavanagh, et al., "Access to lifesaving medical resources," (2020), 1736.

[123] Elijah Songok, "A locally sustainable approach to COVID-19 testing in Africa," *The Lancet Microbe*, (September, 2020), DOI: https://doi.org/10.1016/S2666-5247(20)30118-1.

North. Even that funding has come under scrutiny, suspicion and allegation of theft, as previously highlighted with the major IFIs funding to Kenya.

Testing: Prohibitively Costly and Unavailable

Similar to the cost of quarantine challenge, COVID-19 testing is a pricey affair. For tests besides those performed by the government for free within designated hotspots, cost ranges anywhere from US$100 to US$200 or more, a decidedly "difficult undertaking in a society where more than 40% of the population survives on less than US$2 (Kshs. 216.31)."[124] Unlike the case in other countries, where the cost of COVID-19 testing has either been made good by the government (e.g., the US or the UK) or included in health insurance (e.g., Turkey), Kenya's National Hospital Insurance Fund (NHIF) has traditionally not covered COVID-19 testing. The health sector altogether speaks to "inadequately resourced health systems."[125] COVID-19 has also exposed the folly of the government's inability to see through its commitment to the Abuja Declaration, which pledged to increase the budget allocation to an annual average of 15% of all expenditures. Neither is the country anywhere close to achieving universal health care, unless it borrows a leaf from those that declare victory anyway.

With the sustained emphasis on the role of testing, and the increased production of testing kits around the world, the relative cost of each test has decreased. However, a decrease does not necessarily mean affordability. If the cost of the RT-PCR COVID-19 test required before entering Tanzania, a late entrant into the testing regimen, is anything to go by, the US$25 (Kshs. 2,500) cost is still 10X the average daily income of a near-majority of Kenyans.[126] Beyond testing kits, it is evident that Global Supply Chains are strained to near breaking point, but one surmises that the government cannot possibly plan for

---

[124] Polet Njeri Ouma, Abednego Nzyuko Masai, and Israel Nyaburi Nyadera, "Health coverage and what Kenya can learn from the COVID-19 pandemic," *Journal of Global Health*, vol. 10, No. (2020), 3 doi: 10.7189/jogh.10.020362.

[125] Harison Lagat, Monisha Sharma, Edward Kariithi, George Otieno, David Katz, Sarah Masyuko, Mary Mugambi, Beatrice Wamuti, Bryan Weiner and Carey Farquhar, "Impact of the COVID-19 Pandemic on HIV Testing and Assisted Partner Notification Services, Western Kenya," *AIDS and Behavior*, vol. 24, (2020): 3010–3013, https://doi.org/10.1007/s10461-020-02938-7.

[126] OSAC, "Health Alert: Dar es Salaam (Tanzania), Change in Entry Requirements Due to COVID-19," *Overseas Security Advisory Council, Bureau of Diplomatic Security, U.S. Department of State*, 5th May, 2021, https://www.osac.gov/Content/Report/0b5edea9-2158-43e5-a2b6-1b83766efd6b.

what it cannot see (how many people are infected, where community spread is rapidly increasing or whether testing attitudes have changed among the population etc.) The notion that there can be any alternative, or short-cut to widespread testing, promises to be a mirage on the now 600-day-long road to combating the pandemic.

Testing and Stigma

There are other non-structural, more socially-oriented challenges to COVID-19 testing. Since COVID-19 attracts stigma comparable to that associated with HIV/AIDS, even testing for COVID-19, outside of travel requirements is viewed with immense suspicion. Thus, even when one is unwell and may have contracted COVID-19, they are much more likely to use home remedies than get tested in approved testing facilities. Further, they will likely resort to home care rather than structured medical care, in part too due to the high cost of care and the decrease in number of hospitals attending to the 'regular' illnesses. Hospital and testing center infrastructure also magnifies the potential for stigma.

Overcrowding at most health facilities requires future patients to queue out in the open. Anyone seen approaching a COVID-19 testing site, or designated COVID-19 hospital especially in rural and semi-urban communities where greater social interactions exist, will most likely be the subject of speculation and COVID-19 gossip, whether infected or not. Most Kenyan elites and leaders who get tested for COVID-19 do so in privacy, unlike in other countries where public testing has served as 'confidence-building' measures. At the same time, the experiences of elites such as Raila Odinga, who contracted COVID-19 and recovered, was important in sending a message regarding hospitalization, care and the need to take the pandemic seriously.

Anyone traversing the streets of Kenya in the age of COVID, chin-masks, no-social-distancing, no-testing and 'new normal' will likely be skeptical if COVID-19 really exists. However, one of the most glaring holes in establishing the spread of COVID-19 exists in the absence of data on, or widespread anti-body testing regimes, often referred to as 'seroprevalence.' Per CDC, "a seroprevalence survey uses antibody tests to estimate the percentage of people in a population who have antibodies against SARS-CoV-2. This can tell us how many people in a specific population may have been previously infected with SARS-CoV-2."[127] The record is not all bleak: seroprevalence tests have been conducted, but they are nowhere near adequate, and even those that have been done show a need for *more,* not less. For instance, in September 2020, the measured seroprevalence around the country was 9.1% but higher in Nairobi, in the double digits.[128]

Failing the Test? Serosurveys and Seroprevalence

Other findings point to more widespread infection and recovery around the country. The latter is inferred from the numbers of those in hospital care, ICUs and HDUs. Paradoxically, one might argue that the home care system is working extremely well. Still, a further, seroprevalence study in Nairobi in October 2020 seroprevalence estimated a 42.3% higher incidence and recovery from COVID-19 among transport workers – specifically, truck drivers and their assistants – than the rest of the population.[129] The positivity rate on October 22 was 15.9%.[130]

Whereas transportation crews can be seen to have more face-to-face interactions with the public thus significantly increasing their level of risk of contracting COVID-19, there no specific evidence suggests, globally or nationally, that they are more vulnerable in a way that explains the higher infection and recovery rates. The 43% seroprevalence rate is troubling, and indicative of the higher COVID-19 community spread. The head of Africa's CDC makes this very point, arguing that from a separate serosurvey "study (measuring the occurrence of SARS-CoV-2 antibodies) of blood donors in Kenya" suggests that the actual infection number "translates to ~2.2 million

---

[127] CDC, "What COVID-19 Seroprevalence Surveys Can Tell Us," *The US Centers for Disease Control and Prevention*, Updated July 8, 2020, https://www.cdc.gov/coronavirus/2019-ncov/covid-data/seroprevalance-surveys-tell-us.html.

[128] M. O. Ifedayo, et al., "Temporal trends of SARS-CoV-2 seroprevalence in transfusion blood donors during the first wave of the COVID-19 epidemic in Kenya," *medRxiv* (2021) doi: https://doi.org/10.1101/2021.02.09.21251404.

[129] E. Wangeci Kagucia, et al., "Seroprevalence of anti-SARS-CoV-2 IgG antibodies among truck drivers and assistants in Kenya," *medXRiv* (February, 2021), doi: https://doi.org/10.1101/2021.02.12.21251294.

[130] NERC, "Update on COVID-19 in the Country and Response Measures, as at April 22, 2021," Day 402, Brief No. 394 (Press Statements), Ministry of Health's National Emergency Response Committee, https://www.health.go.ke/wp-content/uploads/2021/04/NERC-MOH-CS-COVID-UPDATE-22.4.2021.pdf.

total possible infections compared with the reported 77,585 infections in the country as of 23 November 2020."[131]

There is a potentially more nefarious and unflattering explanation of the poor levels of testing for COVID-19, or the limited testing and release of seroprevalence data: what you don't know cannot hurt you. The Kenyan government's initial re/actions to COVID-19 were significantly out of proportion with the level of threat that existed at the time. Even though there were many platitudes and promises of action against 'rogue' officers who were 'violating' citizens' 'human rights' after the debacle of the public floggings two hours before curfew, it was clear that government agents had gone far beyond what was necessary to contain the pandemic. If the government's testing consistently produces very low case counts, and evidence elsewhere suggests that the infection and recovery rates are higher,[132] one has to consider plausible inconsistencies in the numbers and narratives.

If the government was not testing enough, or knew that the discrepancy existed between figures provided to the public and the extent of the contagion, what purpose then would it serve, to continue to alarm the public by suggesting that COVID-19 was running rampant – especially considering that the elites in government were not tempering their conduct, like they were asking the rest of the nation to do? Not testing enough, or suppressing the test statistics, neither of which are alleged here, would be served by the practice of reporting few numbers. Of course, the old POTUS '45 argument suggesting that testing produces more cases, and whose argument mirrors the notion that not testing shows lower levels of infection, is unsupported by the facts.

One cannot find that which does not exist, no matter how much they test or don't, can be applied without actually articulating it. By merely not testing, or testing minimally and reporting few cases, the impression is one of a pandemic not spreading or under control.[133] Thus, although both testing and the seroprevalence data and medical records analysis has been quite woeful, and potentially mis-paints the actual COVID-19 situation on the ground in Kenya and in most of Africa, there exists a puzzle (or many puzzles) as to Africa's COVID-19 numbers and outcomes that continues to confound even those in charge. With a case count of 4.5 million and ~106,000 deaths as of

---

[131] Justin M. Maeda and John N. Nkengasong, "The puzzle of the COVID-19 pandemic in Africa," *Science*, Vol. 371, No. 6524 (Jan. 2021), 27-28, doi: 10.1126/science.abf8832.

[132] Maeda and Nkengasong, "The puzzle of the COVID-19 pandemic in Africa," (2021).

[133] Charles Ornstein and Ash Ngu, "No, President Trump, Testing Is Not Causing Case Counts to Rise. The Virus Is Just Spreading Faster," *ProPublica – Coronavirus*, June 25, 2020, https://www.propublica.org/article/state-coronavirus-data-doesnt-support-trumps-misleading-testing-claims.

July 16th, 2021, this represented 2.38% of the 188 million global cases and 2.41% of the global COVID-19 deaths.[134] The African Union's numbers are significantly different, reporting a cumulative 6.13 million cases, 155,502 deaths and almost 5.5 million recoveries.[135]

Even with these statistics, Africa, with its 14 percent of the global population, still accounts for 3.26% of the total cases and 3.8% of global COVID-19 deaths. Compared to the rest of the world, Africa's deaths are higher than world average (deaths over cases), which stands at 2.23%.[136] Notwithstanding, and considering "the continent's overstrained and weak health systems, inadequate financing of health care, paucity in human resources, and challenges posed by existing endemic diseases—including HIV, tuberculosis, and malaria" (in Moeda and Nkengasong's words), the anticipation and prediction that up to 70 million Africans, or almost 6% of the continent would become infected with SARS-CoV-2, has not borne out.[137]

Vaccines and Their Controversies

As important as testing, social-distancing, masks, quarantines, flu shots and proper diet are, the most potent strategy that has seen life return back from 'new normal' to 'almost-old normal' is vaccines. But even as some countries have vaccinated most of their citizens (even in the face of vaccine hesitancy), while some countries have vaccinated *almost none* of their citizens. COVID-19 vaccines are, and have been surrounded by controversy of biblical magnitude: from their development to the speed with which they were tested, to whether Africans were being used as guinea pigs in clinical trials, to availability (who gets what, when) to their administration (in Kenya, the gap between the first and second doses has been – eternity) to opting out of vaccinations due to Evangelical and Catholic Church-driven, religious and moral objections. Even the mRNA technology that creates a fake protein that mimics COVID-19 and is then introduced to the body to encourage formation

---

[134] WHO Africa, "Coronavirus (COVID-19)," *World Health Organization*, Updated July 16th, 2021, https://www.afro.who.int/health-topics/coronavirus-covid-190.

[135] The African Union, (Africa CDC), "Coronavirus Disease 2019 (COVID-19) – Africa CDC COVID-19 Dashboard," *Africa Centres for Disease Control and Prevention* (Africa CDC), July 16th, 2021, https://africacdc.org/covid-19/.

[136] Maeda and Nkengasong, "The puzzle of the COVID-19 pandemic in Africa," (2021).

[137] Maeda and Nkengasong, "The puzzle of the COVID-19 pandemic in Africa," (2021).

of antibodies has been suspected of being fitted with Bill Gates' people-tracking microchips.

The general, scientific consensus on most vaccines, and specifically, the (new) COVID-19 vaccines, is that they are safe and effective, when they are available and taken. Granted, they occasionally have side-effects, but so does most of the medication that is available to most people. Vaccinated persons have been known to experience the so-called 'breakthrough infections,' while the effectiveness of the vaccines has been statistically estimated at anywhere from the 50% range to 98% range. It is especially important to consider the statistical implication of vaccines that are not 100% successful in stopping infection: if they are 95% effective, that implies that out of 100 persons who get vaccinated, 5 can still get infected and sick, notwithstanding being vaccinated. There has been about as much ado about the effectiveness of COVID-19 vaccines as what is in them, but it is perhaps useful to examine the record on other vaccines that have procured less controversy – at least, less than that of COVID-19: the flu vaccine.

Before COVID-19: Thinking About Influenza Viruses

COVID-19 is a respiratory illness, a form of influenza. There are, and have been may types, some with widespread transmission and lethality, and others less so (if one considers SARs and MERS). The exact mortality rate from the flu virus in Kenya remains uncertain, and the data is spotty, if and where it exists. But many scholars suggest that influenza infections remain "a major cause of hospitalizations and deaths every year in Kenya."[138] Common attitudes among Kenyans suggest that 'nobody dies from the flu,' but it is also clear that there are different illnesses that sometimes mimic the flu. For instance, the US CDC advises of the existence of "many other viruses besides flu viruses that can result in flu-like illness (also known as influenza-like illness or "ILI") that spread during the flu season.

These non-flu viruses include rhinovirus (one cause of the "common cold") and respiratory syncytial virus (RSV)."[139] Rather unfortunately, there

---

[138] Duncan Mwangangi Matheka, Jolynne Mokaya and Marybeth Maritim, "Overview of influenza virus infections in Kenya: past, present and future," *The Pan African Medical Journal*, vol. 14, No. 138 (2013), doi: 10.11604/pamj.2013.14.138.2612.

[139] US CDC, "Vaccine Effectiveness: How Well Do the Flu Vaccines Work? Questions & Answers," *The US Centers for Disease Control and Prevention, National Center for*

is not a substantial number of studies and analysis on the kinds of vectors that bring Kenyans to hospital. Some tropical diseases regularly mimic others, and the tendency to favor home remedies makes research into these causes challenging. The potential impact of climatic and other conditions may influence whether a region is more prone to the flu (e.g., the fall/winter flu occurrence in the US). In most of tropical Africa, the common cold, Asthmas and other respiratory issues are likely to mask illnesses that might be the flu. On the other hand, if 'the flu never killed anyone,' Kenyans would be much more likely to then either self-medicate, or use the more common home cures. But neither did COVID-19, until it was diagnosed and its impact made evident.

Even when the flu has been identified as a vector in Kenya, it is unclear if doctors and health-care providers and labs are diagnosing correctly the 'current' strain of the flu, which is often different from the strains manifesting during previous years. As such, if one is testing for a previous (year) strain of the seasonal flu, rather than the (possible current strain, the likelihood of reporting fewer infections by missing the newer strain is high. Still: for the years 2010 to 2018 (excepting 2017), the computed number of flu deaths in Kenya were as follows: ~500, 1,900; 2,000; 500; 1,000; 4,000 and 2,000.[140] It is unclear if flu viruses present across the world, but everywhere, physicians encourage uptake of the flu vaccine, impacting determination of its rate of effectiveness.

That said, according to the CDC's *Morbidity and Mortality Weekly Report*, the 2019-2020 seasonal influenza vaccine was 45% effective against influenza A and B. Specifically, the vaccine was adjudged to be over 50% effective against B/Victoria viruses and 37% against influenza A(H1N1); combined, it produced the 45% effectiveness rate.[141] That explains part of the continued emphasis on getting flu shots,[142] to prevent against *flu* viruses, *despite* the effectiveness that is clearly *lower* than any COVID-19 vaccine

---

Immunization and Respiratory Diseases (NCIRD), Page last reviewed: May 6, 2021, https://www.cdc.gov/flu/vaccines-work/vaccineeffect.htm.

[140] Jeanette Dawa, Gideon O. Emukule, Edwine Barasa, Marc Alain Widdowson, Omu Anzala, Edwin van Leeuwen, Marc Baguelin, Sandra S. Chaves and Rosalind M. Eggo, "Seasonal influenza vaccination in Kenya: an economic evaluation using dynamic transmission modelling," *BMC Medicine*, vol 18, No. 223 (2020), https://doi.org/10.1186/s12916-020-01687-7.

[141] CDC Kenya, "Annual Report 2018," *The Centers for Disease Control and Prevention – Kenya*, 2018, https://www.cdc.gov/globalhealth/countries/kenya/reports/pdf/kenya-annual-report-2018-508.pdf.

[142] AAFP, "CDC Releases Interim Flu Vaccine Effectiveness Report," *The American Academy of Family Physicians*, July 2021, https://www.aafp.org/news/health-of-the-public/20200226interimfluve.html.

currently being offered. In fact, one ought to be puzzled by the COVID-19 vaccine hesitancy, considering the alternative statistic. The CDC reports 39 million illnesses in the 2019–2020 flu season, 18 million as visiting a medical provider, 400,000 hospitalizations and 22,000 deaths – decidedly lower than the 600,000 US and 4,000+ Kenyan COVID-19 deaths. Still, less attention is paid to the flu, its vaccines, mortality rates, vaccine production speed, effectiveness – than COVID-19.

The CDC data is further generous in highlighting the impact of the vaccine. It argues that they "prevented an estimated 7.5 million influenza illnesses, 3.7 million influenza-associated medical visits, 105,000 influenza-associated hospitalizations, and 6,300 influenza-associated deaths."[143] To recap: while surveillance of influenza, infections, uptake of vaccines and related matters is less robust in Kenya, it is clear that (especially flu) vaccines help prevent illness, hospitalizations and deaths, *even when they have a lower efficacy rate* than what might be ideal but unavailable. It is clear too, that considering that SARS-CoV-2 is a flu virus, one could surmise that the reality of much higher efficacy rates and the evidence from vaccines to combat other respiratory and specifically influenza viruses ought to have some significance in the treatment and management of COVID-19.

Why Vaccine Hesitancy? Considering Attenuated Viruses

One of the consequences of the pandemic was that, with restrictions in movement and a slowdown, indeed near halt of most daily and economic activity, almost everyone was essentially confined in place, with nothing to do. That left everyone with little to do other than to be glued to TV and other sources of news, information, misinformation and disinformation. The global nature of the COVID-19 induced inertia implicated the world in following the progress (or lack thereof): of lockdowns, shut-downs, masks, supplies scrambles, lines, curfews and other outcomes of the pandemic.

It also witnessed the rush (or the slow march, depending) towards developing a vaccine, testing it through multiple and diverse pharmaceutical companies' clinical trials, emergency approvals and even with some, the final

143 |US CDC, "Estimated Influenza Illnesses, Medical visits, and Hospitalizations Averted by Vaccination in the United States — 2019–2020 Influenza Season," The US Centers for Disease Control and Prevention, National Center for Immunization and Respiratory Diseases (NCIRD), Page last reviewed: October 6, 2020, https://www.cdc.gov/flu/about/burden-averted/2019-2020.htm.

approval. The public was also transfixed by the media offerings, and became quite well versed with percentages, efficacy, side-effects, arguably, pseudo-knowledge on mRNA, DNA and RNA, scientific terms such as inactivated, attenuated or recombinant vaccine development technologies, and could now point to the several individuals who experienced significant side effects and occasionally death which, in any other medication, would have seemed less threatening to public health.

The most puzzling element of this 'vaccine rejection' and hesitancy was the logical inconsistency with other medical decisions that individuals accept and do, without the same level of scrutiny. For example, as the rumors and suspicion continue(s)(d) to swirl around the various COVID-19 vaccines that were going to be available in Kenya, the Ministry of Health and UNICEF started conducting a nationwide, highly publicized campaign to vaccinate under-5 year old children against polio, another viral disease with debilitating, even fatal consequences for those who develop the full form of the disease. While this discussion in no way asserts any correlation or comparison with the COVID-19 virus, the oral polio vaccine (OPV) that is generally used in Kenya and in most of the other African countries, is a "live-virus vaccine, which [in its development] involved using a weakened form of the polio virus to stimulate antibodies."[144]

The development of the polio vaccine also used testing on monkeys, which seems to be one of the most significant objections to COVID-19 vaccines, never mind the reality that the practice is wide-spread across science. The ultimate formula of the OPV version "consists of three live attenuated Sabin poliovirus strains."[145] One proposes that the potential apprehension and rejection of the COVID-19 vaccine might stem from in-depth knowledge of the virus type, such as is known about polio, but the reality is much different. If Kenyans were aware of the constituent elements of the polio vaccine, or of many other vaccines that are made in the same way, would they still allow their children to have the vaccines considering the attenuated viruses but juxtaposed against the clear benefits accruing?

---

[144] Carl Kurlander and Randy P. Juhl, "Lessons from how the polio vaccine went from the lab to the public that Americans can learn from today," *American Society For Biochemistry And Molecular Biology*, Sept. 26, 2020, https://www.asbmb.org/asbmb-today/science/092620/lessons-from-how-the-polio-vaccine-went-from-the-l.

[145] Anda Baicus, "History of polio vaccination," *World Journal of Virology* vol. 12; No. 1 (4) (2012): 108–114. doi: 10.5501/wjv.v1.i4.108.

Understanding, Sharing the Science behind Vaccines

As noted, vaccines have, particularly during the age of COVID-19, become one of the most hotly contested issues in Kenya and even in the Global North, not because everyone understands the science behind them, or how they – especially with the mRNA versus traditional viruses work. One of persistent and lingering controversies arises from the proposition that some vaccines have been made using stem-cells that are extracted from pregnancies not carried to term. The latter is especially a contested issue, but less so than outright abortion itself. Globally, it is estimated that there are about 42 million abortions annually. Of these, 20 million are in unsafe conditions, often resulting in needless deaths.

Occasionally, fetal tissue and stem cells from those abortions are used to develop vaccines – a concession even the pharma industry has made. In a country that considers itself secular, but where Christianity is almost state-sanctioned, the paradox of church-versus-abortion is most interesting. Churches assert the moral high ground in matters of life, faith, morality and as such, abortion is a hot-button issue, to the extent that even the Catholic Church's opposition to the use of contraception for family planning is well known. It is therefore surprising that there are, on average, about half a million abortions annually (based on data from 2012), an abortion rate of 48 per 1,000 women aged 15-49 with 30 of the 48 abortions being induced.[146]

Even without understanding stem cells or how the science works, the notion that aborted fetuses are harvested to use in the development of COVID-19 and other vaccines has become a hot-button issue in Kenya as well as around the world. Into this controversy stepped the Kenyan Catholic Church, with some Evangelical and Protestant churches chiming in. Institutions, whether they be government, private or international, can offer counterpoints to the legal positions that allow for the use of contentious technology and processes, giving cover to the organizations using them. At the same time, legal positions do not necessarily resolve the contestation surrounding legality versus morality.

One of the contentious issues revolving around vaccines is the use of stem cells, and whether if they are derived from fetuses not brought to term, constitutes of using and supporting 'abortion.' With reference to whether an

---

146 _____ "Incidence and Complications of Unsafe Abortion in Kenya: Key Findings of a National Study," (Nairobi, Kenya: African Population and Health Research Center, Ministry of Health, Kenya, IPAS, and Guttmacher Institute, 2013), https://www.guttmacher.org/sites/default/files/report_pdf/abortion-in-kenya.pdf.

aborted fetus is alive and a human, and at which point life begins so that an abortion equates to murder, has attracted the opinion of the U.S. Supreme Court. Despite *Roe v. Wade,* SCOTUS has ruled "that a fetus is not a person under the terms of the 14th Amendment to the US Constitution but [...] the state had an interest in protecting the life of a fetus after viability."[147] The definition of who is human, or when life begins (biblically, after conception; medically, likely after 'viability' of a fetus) has both allowed drug companies to use fetal tissue to develop some traditional vaccines but also find ways to engineer vaccines that simulate the function of traditional vaccines.

COVID-19 Vaccines, Availability and Vaccine Nationalism

A most interesting, albeit tragic phenomenon has manifested and expanded the schism between the so-called Global North and the Global South. The funding, and scientific discoveries, breakthroughs and administration of COVID-19 vaccines were more robust in the Global North, leading to several countries developing the first COVID-19 vaccines. However, despite the protestations of not trusting the sources of the vaccines (i.e., western nations, a healthy skepticism grounded in their experiences), being made test subjects for a new, probably detrimental vaccine, and being vaccine guinea pigs, the uptake of vaccines in Africa (where they are available) remains significantly diminished.

Vaccine nationalism is generally considered to be the practice of especially developed nations with the wherewithal to research, develop and manufacture especially vaccines, then making available those vaccines to their nationals first, before sale or distribution elsewhere. Essentially, "as countries develop a vaccine, their populations would get first access to it based on their initial investments; once these countries have immunised their populations sufficiently, they would then help international institutions such as the WHO and the UN in the distribution and uptake of the vaccine in all other countries which may have missed out initially."[148]

---

[147] Niranjan Bhattacharya and Phillip Stubblefield, "Of Bioethics, Stem Cells, and Tissue Transplants," In Niranjan Bhattacharya and Phillip Stubblefield, Eds., *Human Fetal Tissue Transplantation*, (London: Springer, 2013), 447.

[148] Marco Hafner, Erez Yerushalmi, Clement Fays, Eliane Dufresne and Christian van Stolk, "Practical implications of "vaccine nationalism": A short-sighted and risky approach in response to COVID-19," *RAND Europe, Research Paper* No. 124, (2020), http://hdl.handle.net/10419/232250] pp. 1.

When nations "take a 'my nation first' approach, where each country solely protects its own interest and competes against others for the initially limited supply of vaccines,"[149] this is often considered 'vaccine nationalism.' The US' perspective when the pandemic first emerged is an excellent articulation of this phenomenon. They "compared the global allocation of vaccines [...] to oxygen masks dropping inside a depressurizing airplane. 'You put on your own first, and then we want to help others as quickly as possible,'"[150] but perhaps forgetting that wearing an oxygen mask in a plane headed for a crash is absolutely unhelpful in the overall outcome.

Different strategies exist, by which countries leverage what then becomes tagged as 'vaccine nationalism.' For example, "some wealthy nations have secured more than 2 billion doses of potential future COVID-19 vaccines using APAs (advance purchase agreements)."[151] But vaccine nationalism is not an entirely new phenomenon. A lot of scholars note that for example, during the 2009 H1N1 (swine flu) vaccine, there was a significant use of APAs, committing 56% of flu vaccines for the years, most of them with industrialized countries.[152] Then, vaccine makers such as Sanofi, GlaxoSmithKline (GSK), Novartis and others, despite the WHO's efforts, committed to produce vaccines for the developed economies, and only about 10% to global health organizations.[153]

For the COVID-19 pandemic, the COVAX partnership was intended to make COVID-19 vaccines available for distribution. It has been unable to secure significant numbers of doses, given the focus of leading economies on own citizens. Although proponents and supporters of nationalist approaches might argue that every nation that has the resources - intellectual, monetary, capacity - ought to benefit from those resources and their application to the search for a vaccine, such arguments fail to appreciate the very nature of the virus and the pandemic.

---

149 Hafner, "Practical Implications," (2020), 1.

150 Thomas J. Bollyky and Chad P. Bown, "The Tragedy of Vaccine Nationalism: Only Cooperation Can End the Pandemic," *Foreign Affairs*, Vol. 99, (Sept./October 2020), 96, https://www.foreignaffairs.com/articles/united-states/2020-07-27/vaccine-nationalism-pandemic.

151 Alexandra L. Phelan, Mark Eccleston-Turner, Michelle Rourke, Allan Maleche, and Chenguang Wang, "Legal agreements: barriers and enablers to global equitable COVID-19 vaccine access," *The Lancet,* vol. 396, no. 10254 (2020), 800. https://doi.org/10.1016/S0140-6736(20)31873-0.

152 Phelan et al., "Legal Agreements," (2020), 800.

153 Abbas, Muhammad Zaheer "Practical implications of 'vaccine nationalism:' A short-sighted and risky approach in response to COVID-19," *Research Paper No. 124*, (2020), South Centre, Geneva.

As long as people breathe and interact with others, vaccinating only part of the world, be they countries, cities, principalities or whichever unit, will likely be insufficient. This was seen in India's case: as the delta variant surged and funeral pyres burned day in day out, the virus was spreading to the US and the UK, which have seen some of the highest vaccination rates. Indeed, some scholars are outright scathing with their assessment of the practice, holding that "this self-centred political behaviour of leaving others behind is short-sighted, potentially risky, morally indefensible, and practically inefficient in containing the pandemic."[154]

Even beyond the argument of the role of the wealthier nations' contribution to global poverty especially in LMICs and LDCs, there are issues with vaccine nationalism. Some accounts present it as "neither ethically justified, nor even in rich countries' long-term self-interest. No one deserves the luck of their birth and few have much control over their country of residence."[155] It is also seen as akin to violation of common standards of decency and human rights; "vaccine nationalism fails to respect basic human rights and the people who have them."[156]

Beyond the question of patents and whether major drug manufacturers should share the vaccine technology [in the interest of humanity], the capacity to produce vaccines, in terms of the sheer volumes and numbers, has been lagging. Estimates suggest that at "current global vaccination rates of roughly 6.7 million doses per day translate to achieving herd immunity (70 to 85% of the population having received a two-dose vaccine) in approximately 4.6 years."[157] Vaccine nationalism led to increasing backlash and calls for equitable distribution of the vaccines, whenever they became available – or at least, when some of the major manufacturers determine to somehow distribute the vaccines equitably. For example, in Germany "Germany is not for sale"[158] started trending, showing that citizens were especially opposed to their companies manufacturing vaccines just for export.

---

[154] Abbas, "Practical implications of 'vaccine nationalism:'' (2020), n.p.

[155] Nicole Hassoun, "Against vaccine nationalism," *Journal of Medical Ethics*, 15 February 2021, http://dx.doi.org/10.1136/medethics-2020-107193.

[156] Hassoun, "Against vaccine nationalism," (2021).

[157] Ingrid T. Katz, Rebecca Weintraub, Linda-Gail Bekker, and Allan M. Brandt, "From Vaccine Nationalism to Vaccine Equity — Finding a Path Forward," *New England Journal of Medicine*, No. 384 (2021): 1281-1283, DOI: 10.1056/NEJMp210361.

[158] Ana Santos Rutschman, "The Reemergence of Vaccine Nationalism" *Georgetown Journal of International Affairs* (online), Saint Louis U. Legal Studies Research Paper No. 2020-16, http://dx.doi.org/10.2139/ssrn.3642858.

However, it also highlighted the complexity of a world now dominated by multinational corporations (MNCs) operating within globalized, global supply chains but with physical locations within countries that then assert the determination to get the vaccines first. This directly opposed the idea that the US "had 'the right to the largest pre-order' of Sanofi COVID-19 vaccines."[159] The nature of this complexity increased, because the US' BARDA (the Biomedical Advanced Research and Development Authority) funded the vaccine development, and as such, the US government had a fair claim to vaccine development. Vaccine nationalism has had and will continue to procure substantial (mostly negative) impacts on Africa, and especially Kenya.

On July 20th, Kenya announced, that it would begin manufacturing vaccines in short order. Presently, vaccination rates tell a story, and it is unpretty. As of July 2021, less than 2 percent of Kenya's total population had been vaccinated. Although there have been marginal increases in the total number of vaccines administered, these have grown relatively slowly. With the Global North nations starting to consider 'booster shots,' essentially a third vaccine, victims of insufficient vaccines are definitely going to be the likes of Kenya.

While it is the case, that righteous outrage has followed every announcement that the Global North was mostly hoarding vaccines and will prioritize their citizens, this is hardly surprising. A walk into any airport will show these separations: there are counters and queues for citizens, nationals, citizens and nationals of regional states, and then everyone else. Visas and immigration control exist for a reason because countries treat people differently. It ought not to be a surprise, that countries prioritize their citizens. After all, they began doing this even with the ban on movement: for the most part, citizens and residents could return, but non-citizens could not.

The only challenge to the 'vaccine nationalism' approach is that no matter how vaccinated one group, citizens of Global North countries or even the people in one country are, new virus variants and mutations are emerging on near-daily basis. They are aggressive, contagious and do not seem to be deterred by vaccines. Considering that COVID-19 is a global pandemic, one whose incubation period length changes little but whose mutations make it all the more transmissible, African countries, and Kenya, will continue being incubators of new versions, variants and mutations of COVID-19, as long as their citizens and residents do not have access to vaccines, no matter how well

[159] Rutschman, "The Reemergence of Vaccine Nationalism," (2020).

the rest of the world is vaccinated. It is in the self-interest of the countries in the Global North then, to someday, share the vaccines and vaccinate most of the world in less than the 6.7 years, so that COVID-19 has nowhere to incubate and mutate.

Wherefore, Kenya?

For the pacifist that is this author, the war hawk Donald Rumsfeld gets more mention and is the source of more quotes than perhaps one might expect. In one of his memoirs, he is reported to have stated something along the lines of *you go to war with the Army you have – not the Army you might wish you have.*' Notwithstanding his politics or alleged war crimes, he is right. African nations, Kenya included, has had to go to war with the army that it has. Although it bungled some elements of what might be considered the invasion (for example, the quarantine facilities and policies were a fiasco, *designed* to fail or procure bribes), it did attempt to deal with the pandemic with the arsenal it had, not the one it wished it had (testing, vaccines and such).

Besides the quarantine facilities, the government has sourced vaccines from every which supplier that might provide them with the doses. It varied its strategy: when it could not get the second dose vials of the Pfizer or AstraZeneca vaccines, it extended the periods between the first and second doses. When only one type of vaccine was available and it differed from the first dose, the government encouraged mixing, long before the proposal to mix vaccines was even considered or recommended, including by the US CDC and the World Health Organization. When countries had vaccines that they could not use and were at risk of expiry, it procured them and literally gave shots to anyone coming off the streets. Kenya was going to war with the army it had, although there were still failures with the efforts to debunk erroneous information coming off social media, the church and other nefarious sources. If the 15+ million doses are anything to go by, Kenya might yet beat the virus by trusting science.

Chapter 4

Government Institutional and Administrative Responses and Reactions

Abstract

This chapter addresses the responses that have been comported by the government and by its institutions in the country. These include governmental institutions and bureaucracies that deal with issues related to politics (e.g., licensing public political rallies), public health (national government ministry, procurement services and major hospitals), administration and public order (e.g., NGAO, the National Government Administration Officers, County Commissioners, police officers, etc.), among others. The chapter addresses what are considered to be 'administrative responses.' The chapter begins by focusing on the most relevant, official and central legislative and administrative organs, new and existing legislation and especially, use of the 'public order act', which was formulated long before independence. The chapter focuses on how pre-colonial era and one-party era rule governance acts and tools have since been updated and applied by successive governments as a catch-all tool, particularly to disrupt political gatherings, but to also impose rather draconian curfews and lockdowns as the pandemic began taking hold. The chapter highlights the irony between the official government response(s) and elites actions where they hold massive public rallies, versus the stated government policy of lockdowns and social distancing. It also examines the simultaneous politicization of the pandemic while the main law-and-order proponent, the government, was holding mass gatherings to promote the abortive Building Bridges Initiative (BBI), and the consequences of the cross-purposes and self-defeating strategies applied.

Preventing and Committing Injustices: of Government Institutions

Whereas 'government' or 'institutional' responses are not neat titles for any discussion, it is useful to examine those issues that are especially pertinent and directly involve the conduct of citizens (and government officials), that either support or imperil the fight against the pandemic. Included therein are government responses to 'stimuli' so that such responses either support or complicate citizens' lives. One must consider the broad purposes of government and the nature of collective welfare, to determine the extent to which both are fulfilled especially in times of crisis, as COVID-19 surely is. Such responses may include supporting citizens with income measures, as was seen widely in Europe and North America, or failure to do so, leading to such queues as were seen in South Africa. These responses are also more directly felt by citizens, unlike such activities as developing a vaccine for COVID-19, which is usually the province of a few select scientists.

In Kenya's case, some of the expected responses are enshrined in the progressive, 2010 Constitution. However, one must recognize that though the constitution speaks of 'every person' being assumed to have 'the right' to something, especially in African societies, this in no way guarantees that such guarantees are actually realized. Article 43 (1) holds that: "every person has the right: to the highest standard of health, which includes the right to health care services, including reproductive health care; to accessible and adequate housing, and to reasonable standards of sanitation; to be free from hunger, and to have adequate food of acceptable quality; to clean and safe water in adequate quantities; and to education."[160] How have these 'rights' been assured in the age of COVID-19, and particularly within the first 600 days of the pandemic?

As previously noted, the Kenyan government is not quite the Olympic gold medalist as far as the prospect of respecting citizens' rights goes. If police – NGAO officers' conduct – is anything to go by, violation of citizens' rights has been more of the norm than exception. But more than *not beating citizens senseless*, such constitutional provisions as being 'free from hunger' and having 'adequate food of acceptable quality' and 'clean and safe water' ought to be the government's priority particularly when it limits daily and especially economic activities, all in the context of a country that was already in the grip of a famine due to poor rains and poor harvests, locus infestations and other sources of food insecurity. This next section takes a closer look at the broader category of 'government institutional responses' and their outcomes.

---

[160] Republic of Kenya, "Kenya Population Situation Analysis," *National Council for Population and Development (NCPD) and the United Nations Population Fund (UNFPA),* (2013), 99 https://www.unfpa.org/sites/default/files/admin-resource/finalpsa report_0.pdf.

Public Order Responses

In the context of COVID-19 and the issue of public gatherings, before considering the President's, NERC's and NGAO's responses, it is helpful to consider the history of restrictions on public meetings and gatherings in Kenya. Such guidance (or perhaps laws) goes as far back as 1950, even before Kenya attained independence, in 1963. Before independence, it was referred to as the 'Native Authority Ordinance' before it was renamed The Public Order Act. It was "created to enable colonial administrators to limit the number of people who assembled in any one place and to monitor gatherings of people, thereby inhibiting political activity."[161]

The Public Order Act is often read together with The Preservation of Public Security Act, Cap.57 of the Laws of Kenya, and Article 58 of Chapter Four (The Bill of Rights) of Kenya's 2010 Constitution.[162] These two are further supplanted by the Chief's Act, now mutilated beyond the original text.[163] The Act dates back to the colonial era, with Chiefs wielding extraordinary powers even to date; the powers include local administrative matters to include land transfers, out-of-court case settlement, runaway children, murderous neighbors and the like.

Administratively, Chiefs were, and still generally are, familiar with, are known to and know most of the residents of the area in which they serve(d). For a famously non-alphabetic society, at least before the end of colonialism, this knowledge was invaluable. Chiefs knew of associations, movements, familial relations, history, politics, religion, dis/agreements, and topography and generally had their ear to the ground, in ways that especially Europeans could not. This was the case *before,* during colonialism and even in contemporary society. Conversely, perhaps because they were the most visible and closest to their African kith and kin. Chiefs were almost always the most hated level of colonial administration because they took on enforcement of whatever new form of oppressing the colonialists were dreaming up, and generally removed the most direct forms of oppression from the colonialists.

---

[161] Diane Ciekawy, "Constitutional and Legal Reform in the Postcolony of Kenya," *Issue: A Journal of Opinion*, Vol. 25, No. 1, (1997), Commentaries in African Studies: Essays about African Social Change and the Meaning of Our Professional Work (1997), 16-18 https://www.jstor.org/stable/1166240.

[162] Ciekawy, "Constitutional and Legal Reform," (1997).

[163] National Council for Law Reporting "Laws of Kenya: The Chiefs' Act, Chapter 128," *Kenya Law Reports – National Council for Law Reporting, 1998* (rev. 2012), http://extwprlegs1.fao.org/docs/pdf/ken102000.pdf.

That said, there were other colonial administrators such as the Provincial and District Commissioners.[164]

After independence, many countries, and especially Kenya, retained the use of Chiefs. As such, throughout the history of most citizens – from pre-colonial, through colonial, to the post-colonial period, citizens of the territory that is today Kenya, have had chiefs loom large over their lives. Today, a Kenyan seeking most government services – identification cards, burial permits, land transfer and its division, or settling minor disagreements between neighbors – is much more likely to interact with the 'chief' than with any other government bureaucracy or officer. Exceptions are when facing judicial processes; then, they might interact with the police, cells, and courts, particularly presently where NGAO officers are tasked with enforcing curfews, enforcing movement bans, assuring social distance measures are kept and prosecuting offenders.

The 2010 Constitution has been heralded as Kenya's, if not one of the world's most progressive constitutions to date. This comparison is likely linked to the now heavily-mutilated, independence-era Lancaster House Conference constitutional resulting documents.[165] The 2010 Constitution did not cause (m)any fundamental alterations to the structure and authority of the Chief's office. Although Chiefs could not restrict movement or declare a state of emergency,[166] the chief was an enforcer of any such restrictions and emergency provisions. Article 58 has governed when, by whom and how a state of emergency may be declared, extended, rescinded, subjected to validity tests, etc. Whereas the Public Order Act covers an array of prohibitions, Part IV, which covers curfews, curfew orders and curfew restriction orders is especially breathtakingly bold. According to Keguro Macharia in the *New Enquiry* blog of December 20, 2014 in which he reproduces parts of the Public Order Act, item 8(1) reads in its entirety as follows:

---

[164] Sorobea Nyachieo Bogonko, "Colonial Chiefs and African Development in Kenya with Special Reference to Secular Education," *Transafrican Journal of History* 14 (1985): 1-20. http://www.jstor.org/stable/24328515.

[165] E. Njoki Wamai, "Mediating Kenya's post-election violence: from a peace-making to a constitutional moment," In Godwin R. Murunga, Dunkan Okelo and Anders Sjogren, *Kenya: The Struggle for a New Constitutional Order*, (London: Zed Books, 2014).

[166] See, for example, Kenya's independence constitution, Article 69, (1-2); 3(b). H.M. The Queen, UK, "Statutory Instruments 1963 No. 1968 Kenya: The Kenya Independence Order in Council, 1963," The Kenya Gazette - Extraordinary Issue - Kenya Gazette Supplement No. 105, (Legislative Supplement No. 69), 10th December, 1963. http://Kenyalaw.org/kl/fileadmin/pdfdownloads/1963_constitution.pdf.

> The Commissioner of Police or a Provincial Commissioner may, if he considers it necessary in the interests of public order so to do, by order (hereinafter referred to as a curfew order) direct that, within such area (being, in the case of a Provincial Commissioner, within his province) and during such hours as may be specified in the curfew order, every person, or, as the case may be, every member of any class of persons specified in the curfew order, shall, except under and in accordance with the terms and conditions of a written permit granted by an authority or person specified in the curfew order, remain indoors in the premises at which he normally resides, or at such other premises as may be authorized by or under the curfew order.

Among other issues that the Public Order Act controls are 'aliens' (their admission or removal), information (prohibition or control of), property and conscription to the public (or para) military service.[167] The version of the Public Order Act that is current has undergone much iteration. It has been subjected to the rhetoric of eliminating most of the 'colonial-era relics' created solely to oppress the African. It has also been subjected to changes, updates and modifications, including in 1950 (twice), 1958 (twice), 1960 (thrice), 1963, 1964 (thrice), 1965, 1968 and 1997, and proposals have been made to restructure and reauthorize it as recently as 2018 and 2019.[168]

Despite years of discussion and the perception that these were tools developed to facilitate the oppression of Africans by colonial authorities, it has never been evident that the government can give up such useful tools to combat dissent and public gatherings. Historically, these 'restrictions' have been broadly used to address, perhaps suppress, anti-government protest activities. The Kenyan government has had significant experience with such suppressions, all the way from independence, to Kisumu in 1969, the multi-party 'saba-saba' protests in 1990, to many other instances.

Herein lies the context: rarely have these measures been applied and enforced in the context of public health crises, but in fairness, there have not been public health crises with the characteristics of COVID-19. However, tactics used in suppression of political dissent, broadly defined, have been applied in the 'regulation' of movement, during the pandemic, be it the public

[167] United Nations, *The International covenant on civil and political rights (CCPR)*, CCPR/C/KEN/2004/227 (September 2004), United Nations – Human Rights: Office of the High Commissioner (OHCHR).

[168] National Council for Law Reporting "Laws of Kenya – The Public Order Act, Chapter 56," *Kenya Law Reports – National Council for Law Reporting / Attorney General, 2003* (rev. 2009), http://www.kenyalaw.org.

humiliations of citizens sitting on the ground hours before curfews, to being beaten with *'jembe'* sticks, whips, being kicked, up to being shot. The current restrictions on movement and enforcement of social distancing and mask mandates then borrowed liberally from tactics thereof.

Public Order Act as a COVID-19 Containment Strategy

In the first address to the nation on COVID-19 on March 15th, 2020, with case count at just 3, the president laid out a number of 'public order' responses and strategies, relating particularly to the gathering and congregating of individuals and measures to facilitate reduction in congregation. Because of COVID-19's transmission pathways, it was necessary, in Kenya just as elsewhere, to limit the movement and *physical interaction* among individuals, *wherever they congregate.* This included educational institutions (schools, colleges etc.), religious gatherings (in churches, mosques, temples and even traditional settings), social gatherings such as dowry, wedding, funeral and other ceremonies, political rallies and related activities, entertainment venues and activities such as night clubs, and a host of other places and circumstances.

In the president's address, items #3, 4 and 5 covered suspension of all learning based on physical presence in education institutions, closing boarding schools by Friday, 20th March, and encouragement of tele-working for both government and business establishments.[169] Although the initial restrictions were emplaced in periods of 30 days, they have continued to be extended, most often in 30 and 60-day increments, often covering the entire nation but equally, sometimes being limited to specific regions and counties in the country.[170] As of July 25th, a new nationwide curfew was still in place from 10 p.m. to 4 a.m.; however, for 13 'hotspot' counties in western Kenya, the curfew begins at 7 p.m. through 4 a.m. The restrictions imposed on June 29th ought to expire in 60 days, hence around August 28th. However, given the rising number of infections, the upwards-trending, all important positivity rate, the persistence of the more contagious, even deadlier delta variant necessarily required a continuation of the most severe of the mitigation measures, including extension, probably even expansion, of the travel bans and other conditions

---

[169] PSCU. "Address to the Nation on Covid-19, Commonly Known as Coronavirus at Harambee House, Nairobi," *The Briefing Room – the Presidency*, 15th March 2020.

[170] AA.com, "COVID-19: Kenya bans political rallies, extends curfew," *Anadolu Agency – Africa, Latest on Coronavirus outbreak,* April 11th, 2020 https://www.aa.com.tr/en/africa/covid-19-kenya-bans-political-rallies-extends-curfew/2032358#.

imposed on the 13 counties. Such measures continued – with the broader nationwide curfew being in place until finally lifted on October 21st, 2021, a full 20 months since it first went into effect.

The heavily publicized, occasional presidential addresses – usually the setting for extension and expansion of the containment measures – illuminate Kenya's COVID-19 challenges. They also provide insight into why the measures are taken. During the *Fifteenth Presidential Address on the Coronavirus pandemic* on Friday, 26th March, 2021, more than a year after the first COVID-19 cases were diagnosed, the president highlighted the positivity rate (19% on March 22nd, steady at 22%). He articulated the following: “if you test 100 Kenyans for COVID today, 20 will be positive; compared to January this year, when only 2 would have been positive.”[171] Besides the positivity rate indicating significant contagion, the president's comments gave room for other analysis. Considering Kenya was testing a paltry 5,000 people a day (or 9.44-5%), and though extrapolating the numbers risks missing the COVID-19 mark, a 22% positivity rate ought to show that more than 11.5 million (of a 53 million population) may have contracted COVID-19.

Power, Politics and Irony: ‘Wananchi versus Wenye-nchi’

One of the most confounding elements of Kenya's COVID-19 pandemic measures is the daylight between words and deeds. The conduct of regular *wananchi* (citizens) compared with the elites (*wenye-nchi*, 'owners of the country) shows the different approaches to the pandemic. For elites, the blatant disregard for the very COVID-19 mitigation strategies to hold political rallies is staggering. Certainly, no citizen of good standing ever wishes someone else ill (especially COVID-19 illness, karma aside), but nobody stands in the middle of a highway and dares cars speeding by to swerve around them either. Elites’ disregard for COVID-19 public health measures is staggering. The approach and conduct are often justified by exhortations to 'fate' and 'destiny,' and the inability of mortals to change either. *'Ni wendi wa Ngai,'* (*it’s God’s will*), *'Mungu akipenda'* and *'inshallah'* are often invoked to demonstrate man's subordinate station to the gods, and his inability to change his destiny.

---

[171] PSCU, "The Fifteenth [15th] Presidential Address on the Coronavirus Pandemic,” Friday 26th March, 2021, State House (Nairobi), Presidential Strategic Communications Unit (PSCU), (2021), 2 http://ke.china-embassy.org/chn/lsfw/P020210328027906621415.pdf.

Since the political class thrives on adulation by citizens, and it has been quite clear (given political rallies and campaigns, by-elections and similar gatherings, that the threat of a pandemic is insufficient to constrain political ambition or even meetings, there have been an increasing number of elites taking ill, or even passing on, from the disease and its complications. It is both rich and ironic that the pandemic is no respecter of title (ask John Pombe Magufuli) or station in life, and some of the very by-elections in which the political class campaigns and seeks to score political points arose due to vacancies created by COVID-19, or 'rona,' as it is wont to be called.

Within a span of three months and ten days, the country lost two – if regional – leaders. The first was occasioned by the untimely death of the Nyamira Governor John Nyangarama (who died on Friday, 18th December 2020), of COVID-19 complications,[172] while on March 30th, 2021, the president was mourning the death of Paul Koinange, Member of Parliament (MP) of Kiambaa Constituency, who died of COVID-19.[173] Governor Nyangarama was an advocate of his county residents adhering to COVID-19 protocols. He "had been leading campaigns aimed at curbing the virus in his county, urging residents to follow guidelines issued by the government through the Health ministry"[174] but succumbed to COVID-19 after hospitalization. In addition, it is widely suspected, even reported, that other notable figures, including then-serving Matungu MP Justus Murunga (November 15th, in Mumias), died of suspected COVID-19 infections.

The other high-profile elite diagnosed with COVID-19 was one-time Prime Minister, current, and arguably perennial presidential candidate *and* the losing candidate in the 2007, 2013 and 2017 elections and long-time fixture of Kenyan politics, Raila Odinga. As Kenya's *de facto* opposition leader, during a March 2018 meeting with President Kenyatta, they ushered in an era of cooperation between government and the opposition, popularized as the 'handshake.' In the subsequent fog of Kenyan politics, the Building Bridges Initiative (BBI) was touted as the implementation of the 'handshake,' and

---

[172] PSCU, "Governor Nyangarama Was A True Servant Leader, President Kenyatta Says," *Presidential Strategic Communications Unit, State House*, December 18, 2020, https://www.president.go.ke/2020/12/18/governor-nyagarama-was-a-true-servant-leader-president-kenyatta-says/.

[173] PSCU, "President Kenyatta Mourns Kiambaa MP Paul Koinange," *Presidential Strategic Communications Unit*, State House, Nairobi, March 31, 2021, https://www.president.go.ke/2021/03/31/president-kenyatta-mourns-kiambaa-mp-paul-koinange/.

[174] Ruth Mbula, "Nyamira Governor John Nyangarama dies aged 74," *Business Daily (Africa) – Counties*, Friday December 18 2020, https://www.businessdailyafrica.com/bd/news/counties/nyamira-governor-john-nyagarama-dies-aged-74-3232608.

would lead to peace. It saw leaders traversing the country to build support for constitutional changes that would also reform the government and the political landscape, more broadly. The substance of the BBI initiative seemed stuck in first gear, subject to legal and political wrangling, but the so-called 'handshake' resulted in the two leaders traversing the country to promote the benefits of both the 'handshake' and future cooperation.

Even as COVID-19 continued to ravage the country, there were no major changes in the conduct of the 'non-political' activities associated with popularizing the BBI initiative across Kenya. "The politics behind COVID-19 also revealed that the former PM Raila Odinga on Citizen Radio declared that COVID-19 would not 'stop reggae' as he prepared the country for a referendum on BBI proposals."[175] When it was announced that Raila had contracted COVID-19 on 10th March 2021, there was a nation-wide perception that perhaps leaders ought to take more seriously the public health measures the same government was urging citizens to adhere to. It was also especially notable that this was the time when the positivity rate, case counts, deaths and hospitalizations were on the rise. On March 11th 2021, Kenya broke its COVID-19 infections record at 1,829, from 6,239 tested samples.[176] These represented 29.32% positivity rate, one of the highest the country has seen – at least until Omicron obtruded upon the world in late 2021.

Keeping with leaders: it is unclear if those who have succumbed to COVID-19 had been part of the 15 million Kenyans who had at least one dose of COVID-19 shot as of February 2022. But they fell squarely into the 'vulnerable' population especially based on age. But even with such high-profile deaths and illnesses, most interestingly but perhaps also equally recklessly, two months later, during the Madaraka Day (June 1st 2021) celebrations, experts were apprehensive over holding public celebrations, even though reports suggested that only 3,000 would be allowed to attend. But in scenes described as 'crowds nightmare,' it was clear that there was more than 3,000 in attendance, with arguments that "non-adherence to the COVID-19

[175] Saidu Umar Mohammed, Musa Saleh, Aliyu Mohammed Malami and Nafiu Mahmood Alhaji, "Politics of Coronavirus in Africa: An Analysis of Kenya and Nigeria," *IJARIIE*, Vol. 6 No. 3 (2020), 591 https://d1wqtxts1xzle7.cloudfront.net/64046395.

[176] Daily Nation, "Kenya's Raila Odinga in isolation after testing positive for Covid-19," *The East African/News/East Africa*, Friday March 12 2021, https://www.theeastafrican.co.ke/tea/news/east-africa/raila-tests-positive-covid-19-3320452.

protocols during the Madaraka Day celebrations [has also] contributed to the surge in numbers."[177]

It is rightfully a not inconsequential challenge to determine if the conduct of individual leaders contributes to the potential for catching COVID-19. After all, it is not *just* politicians that get COVID-19, or attend the rallies. But, the question of 'signaling' is important. Elites can especially change the narrative, model behavior and promote outcomes that decrease congestion and proclivity to exposure to COVID-19, unlike the examples of President Magufuli, Trump, Bolsonaro and others. The role that elites and leaders play can be illustrated with the approach that the new US president took once he came into office: masking was not a political statement – it was science; COVID-19 was not a hoax, social-distancing measures were important, testing was crucial and therapeutics and vaccines were promoted not as some nefarious, Bill Gates' DNA tracking scheme (one wonders why he didn't do that with PCs – less visible and less suspect), and COVID-19 vaccines and transmission misinformation has been one of the prime targets of governments actively combating the pandemic.

What becomes obvious is that especially given the limited testing, vaccines' scarcity and low uptake of other important therapeutics, the government, elites and leaders ought to utilize every other strategy that is available to them, and to citizens, to reduce the impact of the pandemic, even in the absence of COVID-19 vaccines. That, by definition, ought to require adherence to the best COVID-19 mitigation strategies to be the primary strategy. On the other hand, although rational choice theory outlines the process of arriving at a sound decision by considering their objective(s), choices available, their transitivity, the cost-benefit analysis and ultimately, a decision that benefits the individual the most (this is often the basis for individual rationality).

The more complex question is one of whether there is such thing as collective rationality. "It is not [...] obvious, what principles of rationality should govern the choices and evaluations of society,"[178] particularly given the finding that 'the judgments of each of the individuals are consistent with the principles of logic, while social judgments violate them."[179] Arrow's

---

[177] Rushdie Oudia, "Kenya: Nyanza, Western Counties Brace for the Worst of Covid-19 Wave," Daily Nation, (Nairobi), Wednesday, June 9th, 2021, https://nation.africa/kenya/counties/nyanza-western-brace-for-the-worst-of-covid-wave-3430592.

[178] Daniel M. Hausman, "Philosophy of Economics," In *The Stanford Encyclopedia of Philosophy* (Spring 2021 Edition), Edward N. Zalta (ed.), https://plato.stanford.edu/archives/spr2021/entries/economics/.

[179] Hausman, "Philosophy of Economics," (2021), n.p.

discussion in the 'impossibility theorem' is worth becoming familiar with; he "assumes that both individual preferences and social preferences are complete and transitive and that the method of forming social preferences (or making social choices) issues in some social preference ranking or social choice for any possible profile of individual preferences.[180]

Since social choice-making is a joint activity, there are possibilities for a lack of unanimity, incomplete information, dictatorship over preference for one choice, and the impact of external factors on social-choice making.[181] Paradoxically, the question of what one individual can do to contain the spread of the pandemic approximates the exact opposite of the voting challenge. A rational actor who is interested in voting and is a rational actor ought to find that based on cost-benefit, the reality that "the act of voting itself constitutes a small cost of time and effort," voting does not produce any 'great' outcomes, particularly as there are many others undertaking the same practice, thus making any one individual's actions fairly insignificant.[182] Likewise, one individual, be they an elite, leader or citizen, may not consider that their simple actions, such as going to a public rally, might impact the management of COVID-19. In this, the reality of combating the pandemic might be quite a long one.

One suspects however, that negative outcomes are likely to lead to a re-evaluation of the choices that Kenyan society has made, which seems to be the case in the context of COVID-19. Choices that elites make regarding COVID-19 have not entirely succeeded in eliminating the pandemic. In fact, on the contrary, they have held political rallies and events, some straight up politics with masses in attendance. In instances where the government begins enforcing COVID-19 mitigation measures, the political gatherings have often been (barely) disguised. They often take the form of 'meet the people' tours, ‘forums’, ‘barazas,’ while other leaders have frequently attended religious services and ended up making speeches of political nature an increase in the number of COVID-19 infections usually follows.

Perhaps a more useful approach to consider is another econometrics-originating decision-making strategy, the Pareto Optimum (or Pareto-in/efficient outcomes. The benefit of considering the Pareto frontier (and Pareto Optimum) is that individual decisions based on one's rationality do not have to procure disadvantages; in fact, the possibility of improving one's

---

[180] Hausman, "Philosophy of Economics," (2021), n.p.

[181] Hausman, "Philosophy of Economics," (2021), n.p.

[182] James S. Coleman, *Foundations of Social Theory*, (Cambridge, MA: Harvard University Press, 1990), 289.

situation without diminishing that of the other party or parties can be achieved (for example, virtually attending a church service), while the possibility of other frontier points exists.[183] There are both possibilities of individuals reaching their own individual goals, but also the joint preferences. Attending a church service online therefore can protect an individual and group health and wellbeing, but also facilitate religious participation. As the country continues to deal with the pandemic, it is clear that more needs to be done especially by leaders, to not only set a good example, but to also play their part in eradicating the pandemic.

Public Gatherings: Ironies of Leadership

Some of the most confounding elements of the administrative mitigation strategies were in the choices over what types of public activities and crowd gatherings the government could allow and what it would prohibit. And with good reason: a look at any supermarket in Kenya, or queues for *matatus* in the evenings, or even inside them, will demonstrate that these are probably better vector incubators than churches, religious institutions and even schools. Conversely, the very nature of most religious gatherings is the inclusion of such activities that allow for generation of more amounts of (aerosolized) droplets within crowded spaces, one of COVID-19's favorite methods for transmission. For churches – at any rate, some of them – it is part of the religious (or other practice) to engage in such activities as singing and dancing, hugging, sharing sacraments, wine, etc., all of which provide ample opportunities for the virus to spread. Any cursory Google search for 'super-spreader' will usually include 'church.'

That the aforesaid BBI initiative, and the thinly-disguised political meetings, 'meet-the-people' tours, 'civic-education' types of gatherings, national holiday celebrations, or however else these clearly political gatherings were labeled were frequently aired on TV, in news reports and streamed online. Not only were government officials flouting the bans on political gatherings, they often did so with the barest of COVID-19 mitigation strategies adherence. BBI meetings and gatherings have seen little to no social distancing, loud yelling, unmasked attendees, politicians giving speeches without their masks on (granted, they can be constrictive), but without persistent sanitization of some of the podiums or microphones. Removing

[183] Coleman, *Foundations of Social Theory*, (1990).

masks to speak is especially confounding; *that* is precisely when aerosolized drops are ejected and people around are at highest risk, as shown by church and political meets.

The behavior at some of the public rallies approximated that of most religious gatherings but was tinged with more decorum. The collective *angst* at religious restrictions resonated, though evidence showed clear contagion elsewhere. In an Australian case study, a choir member "had sung from a choir loft, elevated 3.5 m above the congregation, which he entered before and left after the service,"[184] then tested positive for COVID-19, leading to 508 contacts, 434 of whom were tested, with a combined secondary attack rate (SAR) of 2.4% or 12 cases, some sitting up to 14 metres from the 'case patient.'[185] After church services resumed in the US in July 2020, "more than 650 coronavirus cases [...] linked to nearly 40 churches and religious events,"[186] including in Texas, especially after the congregation was allowed to hug. In one church in Blenheim, Canada 31 active COVID-19 cases resulted and 300 others went into quarantine. An epidemiologist described it as the "'quintessential super spreader type event.'"[187]

Anyone watching TV or any of those rallies might have been forgiven for thinking that the only attempt to social distancing was to give the impression that one was adhering to such guidance, rather than for the benefits it procures. The expectation that politicians, when they go on the 'meet/greet-the-people' tours, will 'incentivize' the public by giving away money almost necessarily made it inevitable that citizens would attend the rallies, or whatever they were. Even rational choice would suggest that a Kenyan's individual chances of being diagnosed with COVID-19, with the confirmed cases at 350,000 as of February 2022, in a total population of 54 million, was about 0.61%, while those of dying of COVID-19 calculated on the basis of the whole population, are 0.011% over the two years.

---

[184] Anthea L. Katelaris, Jessica Wells, Penelope Clark, Sophie Norton, Rebecca Rockett, Alicia Arnott, Vitali Sintchenko, Stephen Corbett, and Shopna K. Bag, "Epidemiologic Evidence for Airborne Transmission of SARS-CoV-2 during Church Singing, Australia, 2020," *Emerging Infectious Diseases Journal*, Vol. 27, No. 6 (June 2021), 677-1680. doi:10.3201/eid2706.210465.

[185] Katelaris, ""Epidemiologic Evidence for Airborne Transmission of SARS-CoV-2 (2021), n.p.

[186] Kate Conger, Jack Healy and Lucy Tompkins, "Churches Were Eager to Reopen. Now They Are Confronting Coronavirus Cases, "*The New York Times*, Updated July 10, 2020, https://www.nytimes.com/2020/07/08/us/coronavirus-churches-outbreaks.html.

[187] Jennifer La Grassa, "Epidemiologist says small spaces where people spend lots of time have increase transmission risk," *Canadian Broadcasting Corporation News*, Updated: October 31, 2020, https://www.cbc.ca/news/canada/windsor/covid-19-church-spreader-event-1.5783090.

It therefore meant that going to the rallies in the hope of securing some money was a calculated, and decidedly financially acceptable, if not a worthy risk. And although the causes are disparate, a recent Global Hunger Report ranked Kenya among 40 countries with a score of 23.7 (serious risk of hunger) for over 1.5 million people, 7.5X the total positive COVID-19 cases.[188] Clearly, the risk of getting COVID-19, weighed against the threat of starvation, which is more prescient, or the childhood deaths due to malnutrition and hunger with the "percentage of children younger than 5 years at risk of malnutrition [is] more than 21%"[189] prompts one to take even greater risk, especially in the absence of government nutritional support.

Failing to model behavior that would have provided a modicum of *consistency* in messaging and actions suggests that the government and elites lost both credibility and a chance to actually contain the spread of the pandemic. At the same time, it is imprudent to dismiss all the evidence that shows that even though children are not seriously affected by the pandemic, schools and churches are incubators for the SARS-CoV-2-2 virus, and not closing them risked spreading the pandemic to more vulnerable family members at home. However, what has been lacking is consistency, an 'all-of-the-above' approach so that even political gatherings are not allowed; otherwise, the whole pandemic-fighting strategy, particularly where social distancing is required, is moot.

Corruption and Rent-Seeking

That Kenya is ranked amongst the most corrupt nations in Africa and the world is not worth repeating. At this point, it is even fairly unremarkable, almost as certain as the sunrise. If the six degrees of separation is a true concept, applying the same to corruption in Kenya, from the nexus to the periphery, suggests that corruption has touched *every* Kenyan, or they have been present at a corrupt transaction. It is often at institutional level, but it is also pervasive at the Kshs. 50, 100, 1,000 or other levels, based on the service one is seeking,

[188] Allan Mungai, "Report reveals 1.5 million Kenyans are facing hunger as locusts, COVID bites," Financial Standard, February 25th 2021, https://www.standardmedia.co.ke/business/financial-standard/article/2001404502/report-reveals-15million-kenyans-are-facing-hunger.

[189] Sam Loewenberg, "Breaking the cycle: drought and hunger in Kenya," *The Lancet*, Vol. 383, No. 9922 (March 22, 2014), 1025-1028 (special report) DOI: https://doi.org/10.1016/S0140-6736(14)60492-X.

or the prohibitions one intends to circumvent. Often, graft-seekers create such circumstances as to make bribe-giving *the most logical* course of action. But when it comes to those issues and instances that can be life-threatening, for example paying to get out of quarantine (even if one might be infected with COVID-19), or bribing police or NTSA for an intoxicated driver to get past a checkpoint or for a criminal to go free, the country begins working against its collective interest.

In 2019, TI's Kenya's CPI score was 28 out of a possible total 100 points. It was ranked 137 of 180 countries, scoring below Sub-Saharan Africa's 32 points average and substantially below the global average of 43 points. The gap between Denmark and New Zealand (87) and Kenya is almost 60 points, and even though the (failed) states of Somalia, South Sudan and Syria were lower at 9, 12 and 13 points, Kenya should not be in this company given its fairly long-term political stability.[190] Even more troublingly, the past 10 years have not seen its score budge from anywhere between 25 and 28. It also ranks far below two of its major EAC compatriots such as Rwanda (53) and Tanzania (37), and is tied with Uganda.[191] Data from 2017 shows that 40% of Kenyans reported paying bribes to access government services, with a five year average percentage at 37.[192]

In terms of corruption at institutional level (Perception of Corruption by Institution) 2017 (2013) data shows that 98% perceived police to be corrupt, 68% the legislature, 59% government officials, 29% business executives, 58% judges an magistrates and 15% religious leaders.[193] It is not clear that any of the perceptions have changed since the data collection, particularly given that the advent of social media and more technologically advanced communications equipment has provided occasion to film different individuals proposing, taking or giving bribes. There is some good news though: in 2020, either because of, or in spite of COVID-19, on the TI-CPI ranking, Kenya cracked the 30 score, with 31 points and a 124th global ranking.[194]

---

[190] TI Kenya, "Corruption Perception Index 2019," *Corruption Perception Index*, Nairobi, Kenya, 23rd January 2020, https://tikenya.org/corruption-perceptions-index-2019/.

[191] TI Kenya, "Corruption Perception Index 2019," (2020).

[192] Ourworldindata, "Corruption Perception Index vs. Share of people who have bribed, 2017," *Our World in Data*, Retrieved on 7/28/2021, https://ourworldindata.org/grapher/share-of-people-paying-bribes-vs-corruption-perception.

[193] Ourworldindata, "Perception of Corruption by Institution, World, 2017," *Our World in Data*, https://ourworldindata.org/grapher/perception-of-corruption-by-institution?country.

[194] Transparency International, "Corruption Perceptions Index," *Transparency International*, 2021, https://www.transparency.org/en/cpi/2020/table/ken#.

Most citizens are unlikely to be touched by institutional-level corruption. They are likely to have to give a bribe to low-level government functionaries such as police officers, chiefs, judges, military recruiters, college heads, head teachers and others in these categories, rather than, as an example, multi-million dollar contracts. The vetting of police officers and accounting for their wealth has never been serious on any level. Regarding perception of the seriousness of corruption in the public sector, on a scale of 1-5 (not serious to most serious), Kenya's score was 4.3, approaching the 'very serious problem' category.[195] One surmises that Transparency International has not caught on to the COVID Billionaires' scandal that has captured the imagination of the country during the pandemic.

Corruption in Enforcing COVID-19 Restrictions

Corruption in the Matatu (transport) industry is so rife that it is formulaic. A *matatu* approaches a police road-block. It is waved to a stop. The police officer pretends to go around the vehicle, presumably inspecting it for some unspecified fault. Passing by the driver's door, he – or she – unhooks a Kshs. 50 currency note (or Kshs. 100 note – more on that later) that has been folded and placed under the driver's door latch. It is a barely perceptible, quick exchange, one that leaves the driver with plausible deniability because one can literally see the driver's hands, and affirm that there was no visible exchange, and therefore, it is especially challenging to assert bribery. Additionally, since there are few recording devices, it is exceedingly difficult to procure evidence of wrongdoing, outside of the occasional public relations 'sting' operations.

On occasion, citizen passengers are co-opted by the matatu crew, to help pass the currency note forward to the driver, so that it can be properly 'hooked' in the right place before the Matatu comes to a stop. The transaction is quick, flawless, and repeated at different places along a Matatu's route. The next day, the process begins again, making the entire process especially lucrative for the police especially. For a price, the Matatus will go unmolested for that day. Other victims are usually tractor-trailers, large (and sometimes small) vans, and the occasional private vehicle. Private vehicles can be quite lucrative, especially since if one is unaware of traffic laws and therefore any infractions they may have committed, they are likely to want to minimize the interaction

[195] Ourworldindata, "Average rating of perceived corruption in public sector, 2013," *Our World in Data*, https://ourworldindata.org/grapher/average-rating-of-corruption-perception.

by offering what both parties *know* the police want, but that neither will articulate: ‘road tax.’

Enforcing (or un-enforcing) COVID-19 restrictions has become the newest cash-cow. Since the government asserted that social-distancing measures should be implemented in public transportation, it was necessary to reduce the capacity of passengers in a vehicle, usually by 30%. For the common 14-seater matatu, that meant ten passengers: three per row and one next to the driver. The 25-seater and 33-seater mini-buses also reduced capacity appropriately, although the formula just suggested a one-third reduction. In the context and shape of a matatu, the notion that one could keep six feet (or in Kenya’s context, 1.5 meters) away from another passenger when the matatus have one entry, which also serves as the exit, is impossible. Matatus have quite a lengthy history of flouting government guidelines on practically every road rule invented. As such, exceeding capacity is almost natural. Matatus exceed capacity and thus flout social-distancing rules, but continue operating because they replace the Kshs. 50 note with a Kshs. 100 note, as the new, COVID-19-guideline-flouting ‘road tax.’

This is the quintessential concept expressed in people working against their very own interests, pursuing short-term gains in lieu of helping combat the pandemic. But more than that, and perhaps in a discussion more appropriate to *Bandit Nations* rather than Kenya’s strategies to contain COVID-19, matatus’ behavior then (and continuously) approximates 'fiscal disobedience.' 'Fiscal disobedience' refers to a situation "whereby the legitimacy of regulatory authority is questioned and undermined, matatu workers as infrastructure challenge multiple levels of state and non-state regulation through a variety of practices that blend danger, violence and control with solidarity, reciprocity and redistribution [...] as they navigate dangerous negotiations with the state, the police and vigilante gangs."[196] To possibly contain the spread of the pandemic, the government needs to have control of the matatu sector, and given the momentous task, it is not clear that this is feasible.

Besides the matatu debacle, enforcing mask mandates has been another lucrative source of ‘private equity’ for the police. A single mask is likely to cost Kshs. 10. Not having a mask risks a fine o anywhere from Kshs. 1,000 to Kshs. 20,000. As previously discussed, this almost a quarter of most average Kenyans’ annual income. Being arrested without a mask risks such profound

---

[196] Meghan E. Ference, "‘You will build me’: fiscal disobedience, reciprocity and the dangerous negotiations of redistribution on Nairobi's matatu," *Africa*, Vol. 91, No. 1 (2021), 16-34, DOI: https://doi.org/10.1017/S0001972020000820.

consequences that it is almost inevitable that paying a bribe is the easier route. If one considers arrest (rather than say, a ticket or a citation), spending a night in a cell, crowded, filthy and downright a health hazard, with other suspects who may, or may not have masks (even the arrest and transportation process does not guarantee that social distancing, sanitizing or masks are worn by those arrested) simply paying a Kshs. 500 bribe so as *not* to be arrested is not only in one's self interest, it is rational.

Curfew enforcement was previously alluded to; it initially led to the deaths of tens of Kenyans at the hands of police under the NGAO umbrella. Curfew enforcement continues to be another most lucrative opportunity for law enforcement. Violating curfew, whether during the pandemic or during other times when such curfew has been implemented, can bring unpalatable consequences. These include arrest, detention in police cells, remand in actual jails and prisons under the said atrocious conditions. Just as with masks, it is often prudent, if illegal, to minimize one's exposure and legal jeopardy, for it may extend beyond a night in cells or a fine. A young man arrested for '*masaa mbaya'* (violating rules barring alcohol consumption in clubs beyond 2 a.m.). After his arrest and two-week remand at Naivasha G.K. Prison, he was promptly diagnosed with cholera. Clearly, the long-term cost in resources and health necessitate *not* being arrested, by any means.

A curious practice thrives in Kenya's urban areas, particularly with the almost-reputable clubs, hotels, accommodation spots, and bed-and-breakfast establishments. While they do 'observe' curfew hours (10 p.m. to 4 a.m. as of August 2021), they do so creatively. Any of the customers within the establishment may generally be allowed to stay inside (not that they have a choice, unless they plan on having a run-in with the law). Because police officers can exercise the prerogative to require any business to open for inspection regarding COVID-19 compliance levels, some establishments provide incentive for the law enforcement members – they may drink for free, or actually collect 'COVID-19 curfew taxes' so that there is continued operation by the said establishment. In the event of other law enforcement professionals visiting the establishment, the first group might offer 'guarantees' against any harassment. Clearly, prohibition produces opportunities for law-breaking.

Other forms of corruption are low level, less obvious and even contestable, over whether their classification as 'corruption' is appropriate or justified. Examples include the idea that "this corruption largely takes the form of absenteeism and poor performance among doctors and nurses who are on the public payroll."[197] Good, timely access to care itself is an opportunity for rent-seeking, although accusations against medical professionals who are presumably guided by the Hippocratic Oath; yet Kenya's health system is full of 'quacks' and hacks, capable of injecting water in lieu of vaccines. Determining who gets treatment where, how much it costs and who has priority and payment of hospital costs, even via the NHIF, can imperil the provision of healthcare in unsavory ways. As such, it is not just the police; at every level of provision of services, corruption opportunities manifest.

Other Macro, Policy-Level Interventions

The government also undertook a series of macro-level policy interventions that included budgetary, tax relief, administrative and regulatory actions that positively impacted the well-being of Kenyans. These included a 100% tax relief on those employees making Kshs. 24,000 or less (about US$240 a month), a reduction of the PAYE (Pay As You Earn) (income) tax by 5% from 30% and a similar margin reduction in the Corporation Tax, a 2% reduction in turnover tax rate for SMEs, to 1% and for everyone, a reduction in the Value Added Tax (VAT) from 16% to 14%. Given the job-losses that came about due to the pandemic, loan defaulters would not be listed at the Credit Reference Bureau (CRB) until the economy returned to a better footing and the pandemic was better contained.[198]

Some of the other actions included a temporary elimination and/or reduction of mobile money transaction fees, in line with the president's first Coronavirus address, encouraged banks to refinance loans and relax the repayment terms or postpone due dates, while the Central Bank of Kenya (CBK) cut interest rates and injected money into banks to ensure continuing liquidity.[199] The government also embarked on strategies to increase FDI into the country despite the challenging global environment. The government also

---

[197] Stuti Khema, "An Opportunity to Build Legitimacy and Trust in Public Institutions in the Time of COVID-19," *World Bank Research & Policy Briefs* - World Bank Malaysia Hub, No. 32, (May 4, 2020), 2 https://ssrn.com/abstract=3602352.

[198] Monica K. Kansiime, Justice A. Tambo, Idah Mugambia, Mary Bundi, Augustine Kara, and Charles Owuor, "COVID-19 implications on household income and food security in Kenya and Uganda: Findings from a rapid assessment," *World Development*, Vol. 137 (2021), 2-3 https://doi.org/10.1016/j.worlddev.2020.105199.

[199] IMF, "IMF Country Focus: IMF Loan to Support Economic Recovery in Kenya," *The International Monetary Fund*, March 18, 2021, https://www.imf.org/en/News/Articles/2021/03/17/na031721-imf-loan-to-support-economic-recovery-in-kenya.

obtained loans, grants and deferrals from development partners, multilateral and international institutional donors, the most significant being the World Bank, although in the context of the 'COVID millionaires', this 'reckless' borrowing caused great consternation, calls for greater accountability and even low-level protests by Kenyans.[200]

As previously discussed, the government also engaged in deficit-spending, although again, the debt-to-GDP ratio, or the amount of government debt as a share of the GDP in September 2020 was 68.6%,[201] having climbed from a low of 39.7% in 2010. Given a decline in collected and anticipated revenues, the overall economic conditions and the 8-point economic stimulus programme, government also decreased the allocations to its cabinet departments, departments and state enterprises, by 6.8%. The ministry of health did see a much needed, but subsequently misused 10.3% increase in its allocation over the previous year, while allocations to county governments decreased by 2.3%.[202] The balancing act was unpopular with the county governments, although given the reality of a national pandemic that required an 'all of government' approach, consolidated government actions were more likely to produce better outcomes than piecemeal, County Government-designed strategies.

COVID-19 Meets Kenyan Realities: WFH, *Matatus* etc.

One of the challenges that bedeviled Kenya's efforts to contain the pandemic is the nature of work that most Kenyans perform. As soon as the government suggested teleworking, working from home or working at distance, it became clear that the Kenyan employment condition does not favor anything but in-person work interactions, which decidedly complicated the fight against COVID-19. This arose from a combination of factors. About 40% of Kenya's 53 million works in the agricultural sector, including 70% of rural dwellers;

200 V. Nechifor, E. Ferrari, E. Kihiu, J. Laichena, D. Omanyo, R. Musamali and B. Kiriga, *COVID-19 impacts and short-term economic recovery in Kenya, EUR 30296 EN*, (Publications Office of the European Union, Luxembourg, 2020),14, doi:10.2760/767447, JRC121284.

201 CEIC, "Kenya Government Debt: % of GDP," *2009 - 2020 | Quarterly | % | CEIC Data*, https://www.ceicdata.com/en/indicator/kenya/government-debt--of-nominal-GDP.

202 Boniface Owino, "Kenya's Covid-19 budget: Funding for health and welfare," *Development Initiatives*, 2 July 2020, https://devinit.org/resources/kenyas-covid-19-budget-funding-for-health-and-welfare/.

agriculture accounts for 33% of Kenya's GDP.[203] On its part, the World Bank estimates 21.9% of GDP and 56% of total labor force employed in Agriculture, as well as a 31.4% reduction in poverty as a result of agriculture in the pre-COVID-19 environment.[204] The International Trade Association pegs Kenya's share of the workforce in Agriculture at 40%, 25% of GDP in direct contributions and 27% contribution through linkage with different sectors.[205]

For the most part, those working in agriculture rarely need to travel to work, but another statistic illuminates the challenge for the formal sector. One estimate finds that "over 80 percent of workers are confined to informal jobs, which are typically low pay and low skill."[206] Although it is an inelegant, Euro-centric measurement strategy (for example, that one does not buy furniture from IKEA should not count against those countries that have excellent carpenters); data from the Swiss Institute of Technology (KOF) shows Kenya's economic globalization at an average of 41 points (latest data, 2018), down from a high of 47.29 in 1993. Although a substantive majority of Kenyans being engaged in the agricultural sector, mostly in small scale farming and enterprises and increasingly, agribusiness, those that work in the formal sector, alongside farmers themselves, overwhelmingly use *matatus* to get to places.

Social distancing introduced several inadvertent measures: by decreasing the capacity in matatus, fares went up in an attempt to compensate for the fewer passengers per matatu, which made travel less desirable. Such increases were not untoward; it is a private sector, ruled by the law of the jungle, and anti-trust is just a word. Secondly, by introducing curfews and lockdowns with the kind of beating seen in Mombasa and other 'curfew enforcement deaths' across the country, citizens had incentive to get into matatus, overcrowded or not, consequences be damned. Downsides included possibly catching COVID due to overcrowding. Thirdly, since the matatu sector is also a major employer, capacity reduction meant job losses, and withdrawal of matatus

---

[203] USAID, "Kenya: Agriculture and Food Security – Overview," *USAID*, Last updated: June 03, 2021, https://www.usaid.gov/kenya/agriculture-and-food-security.

[204] The World Bank, "Kenya Economic Update: Transforming Agricultural Productivity to Achieve Food Security for All," *World Bank – IBRD & IDA*, April 2019, https://www.worldbank.org/en/country/kenya/publication/kenya-economic-update-transforming-agricultural-productivity-to-achieve-food-security-for-all.

[205] International Trade Administration, "Kenya - Country Commercial Guide: Agribusiness," *International Trade Administration*, 13th September, 2020, https://www.trade.gov/country-commercial-guides/kenya-agribusiness.

[206] Hannah Timmis, "Jobs in Kenya: Opportunities and Challenges," K4D Helpdesk Report. Brighton, UK: Institute of Development Studies. https://opendocs.ids.ac.uk/opendocs/handle/20.500.12413/13619.

from business, leaving few matatus operating in a socially-distant environment with curfews and lockdowns.

Kenyan firms and government agencies quickly discovered that they were not exactly built, or ready, for tele-working, or working from home, now famously abbreviated as WFH. From a lack of internet connectivity to its high cost and unreliability, to challenges wrought by infrastructure (especially electrical connectivity that is unreliable at best), to high costs of outfitting homes that are often unsuitable to work in, there was no shortage of challenges to tele-working. Some of the other challenges are more structural; for instance, the "exports of digitisable goods in Q2 of 2020 have in fact declined in Thailand, Brazil, Kenya and Mozambique."[207] In the middle of the pandemic, Kenyan firms faced the need to retool for a different business environment. "COVID-19 has also accelerated the urgency for adaptability and transformation across industry and business models, with an estimated 70% of new value being created through digital business models."[208]

Specific to Kenya, "30% of the members in the Kenya Association of manufacturers (KAM) surveyed are aiming to increase online capabilities as a response to the crisis."[209] This is notably an expression of interest in retooling, almost nine months after the pandemic started. This assured that these, and most businesses, were *not* ready before the pandemic. African – and Kenyan – companies are also disadvantaged in the areas of data storage, reliability, usage and broadband speed. This explains why "less than 1% of estimated public cloud services revenue was generated in Africa as of 2018."[210] Although Cloud Management Insider's Cloud Evangelist rudely blames Africa's cloud services challenges on apparent "decades of ignorance and poor basic infrastructure," they point to server location issues (mostly abroad), which raises questions of use and storage of citizens' data elsewhere, or data sovereignty.[211]

Compensation for job losses (income support) was one of the other global strategies to deal with the pandemic. For those who worked in the formal

---

[207] Karismha Banga and Dirk Willem te Velde, "COVID-19 and disruption of the digital economy; evidence from low and middle-income countries," *Overseas Development Institute* – Digital Pathways at Oxford, Paper Series, Paper 7, (December 2020), ii, https://pathwayscommission.bsg.ox.ac.uk/sites/default/files/2021-01/covid-19_and_ disruption_of_the_digital_economy_28jan21.pdf.

[208] Banga and te Velde, "COVID-19 and disruption of the digital economy," (2020), 7.

[209] Banga and te Velde, "COVID-19 and disruption of the digital economy," (2020), 2.

[210] Banga and te Velde, "COVID-19 and disruption of the digital economy," (2020), 13.

[211] Cloud Evangelist, "Why the least tapped market is the next big thing in cloud," *Cloud Management Insider*, October 9th, 2019, https://www.cloudmanagementinsider.com/why-african-market-next-big-thing-in-cloud/.

sector and who lost jobs as a result of the pandemic, in most countries, some form of income support, or income replacement (and in the case of the US, the Paycheck Protection Program) provided economic support to mitigate income loss. African countries did attempt to provide some sort of economic support, although the average amount especially in Sub Saharan Africa was just above 10% and replaced less than 50% of the lost salary in both formal and informal sectors. This compared poorly with South Asia, Europe and Central Asia and North America, where such assistance was above 50% and 60% for the latter two. In Kenya's case, this juxtaposed against stringent application of COVID-19 measures at above 85%.[212]

[212] Michael Danquah, Simone Schotte, and Kunal Sen, "COVID-19 and Employment: Insights from the Sub-Saharan African Experience," *Indian Journal of Labor Economics*, Vol. 63, (2020), 23–30 https://doi.org/10.1007/s41027-020-00251-4.

Chapter 5

Economic Impacts, Governance Implications and Educational Outcomes

Abstract

This chapter examines some of the most significant impacts that have occurred as a result of the COVID-19 pandemic, affecting individuals, firms and government's overall economic production and conditions due to work stoppages, shutdown of businesses and lockdowns in an environment of minimal welfare support. It also touches the impact of the COVID-19 induced economic slowdowns, shutdowns and declining welfare. It begins by detailing how imposition of COVID-19 mitigation measures exacerbated corruption – both institutional (targeting donor and World Bank funding) and petty corruption (targeting the enforcement of face masks, compliance with curfews) and the suspected sale of medical equipment and PPE, as well as vaccines when they became available. It also highlights the additional macro, policy-level interventions and whether they have worked. In terms of education, COVID-19's stoppage of learning has had significant impacts, beginning with the changes in the educational experiences, calendars, content delivery and even school lunches, particularly in the middle of a switch in the education system to the much-derided Competency-based Curriculum (CBC). It proposes that the impacts of interrupted learning experiences will be felt for a long time. The chapter also examines the lessons learnt (or that we should learn) in proofing systems, especially education and attempts at distance education in a state of insufficient infrastructure. The chapter concludes that Kenya's critical government and institutional responses and reactions have fallen significantly short of what is necessary to mitigate COVID-19, and emerge with fairly robust society, education and institutions.

Before COVID-19: The Corruption Pandemic Afflicting Us

Although the major focus of this chapter is not necessarily the corruption that has been so pervasive in the life of the republic, one cannot adequately discuss Kenya's COVID-19 pandemic strategies and management without addressing corruption, at institutional and petty levels. More broadly, the issue of corruption addresses itself to the form and purpose of governance, and to the levels of trust that citizens have in government, the credibility that the government thus enjoys, its ability to command citizen compliance with its directives and the overall outcomes of such interactions. Legitimacy is important, and if citizens perceive government to be less than legitimate, carrying out its agenda, especially around an issue as important as COVID-19 management, can be a great challenge. Legitimacy and ability of government to command the respect of citizens also speaks to the effectiveness of the proposed and implemented strategies. And the issue of corruption is not only pertinent to pandemic management, but to other broader issues impacted by COVID-19. This was also seen in how the government supported (or did not), by economic means (such as income replacement), especially the most marginalized societies, for example individuals living in the informal settlements (or slums). Requiring them to stop work while failing to provide alternative sources of income could only increase poverty. It was poor policy and pandemic management.

Besides the persistent levels of corruption including with embezzlement of funds meant to help the country combat the pandemic and obtain PPE and related resources, government decisions impacted education, through the closure of educational institutions. Education is often considered to be the 'great equalizer,' the most direct path to well-being particularly for the less-resourced in Kenya and many other similar societies. Estimates have shown that the pandemic negatively impacted the provision of education, achievement, retention and even the ability to transition successfully across grades. The sense of equity demands that all Kenyan kids have a fair chance at obtaining education, without disadvantaging some. When schools shut down due to the requirement to eliminate in-person sessions, some schools went ahead and started delivering content online. Given that at the end of certain periods (or grades/classes, e.g., Standard 8 and Form 4) there are national exams, this no doubt disadvantages those children whose families are unable to afford the technology or funding to pay teachers to learn while the other pupils were home under the COVID-19 conditions.

Institutional Corruption Around COVID-19

Institutional-level corruption has been another of the perennial challenges faced by Kenya. During the waning years of the Cold War and in the 1990s, western governments, donors, lenders, development partners and IFIs resorted to suspending aid to Kenya and other African countries due to corruption, among other governance issues. The situation has not changed much even today: eradicating corruption remains one of the conditionalities for most development assistance, aid and foreign direct investment, even though Kenya and other African countries have found other willing funders and development partners in China and more broadly, BRICs. That said, institutional-level corruption in Kenya, as show previously, is rampant, with 98% of respondents labeling the police as corrupt. If 98% was the efficacy rate for the COVID-19 vaccines, everyone would have them.

There are obvious institutional risks to corruption, particularly when the stakes are as high as they are, during a pandemic that is past the 500th day and seems to be *accelerating* in its spread and severity. Some of the 'consequences' of corruption are seen in the health sector and are identified as; "emergency procurement that increases corruption risks; pilfering available supplies, price gouging, and resale on the grey and black markets; [and an] increase in substandard and falsified products entering the market."[213] Corruption can include embezzlement and diversion of resources for private use, hoarding or resale, including those purchased, given or donated for specific purposes.

Kenya has been hit by nearly all types of these corruption incidents. For example, "six million face masks ordered by Germany to protect health workers from the corona virus went missing at an airport in Kenya."[214] Besides the German supplies disappearing as 'magic masks,' later on there was an "alleged disappearance of donations by Chinese philanthropist Jack Ma,[215] therefore reflecting on the historical trend of misappropriation of public health funds and resources."[216] The level of silence around these donations is especially staggering, as is the destructive nature of the diversion of such resources so that they do not reach those most vulnerable to COVID-19 or on the frontlines. But perhaps the most stinging rebuke to the government's handling of the COVID-19 crisis regarding procurement of life-saving PPE,

---

213 Sarah Steingrüber, Monica Kirya, David Jackson and Saul Mullard, "Corruption in the time ofCOVID-19: A double-threat for low income countries," Chr. Michelsen Institute (Norway), U4 Brief, No. 6 (2020), 4. https://www.u4.no/publications/corruption-in-the-time-of-covid-19-a-double-threat-for-low-income-countries.pdf.

214 Steingrüber, et al., "Corruption in the time ofCOVID-19," (2020), 4.

215 Georja Calvin-Smith and Laura Di Biasio, "Billionaire Jack Ma's Covid-19 donations to Kenya go missing," *France 24 - Eye on Africa*, Modified: 03/09/2020, https://www.france 24.com/en/africa/20200903-kenya-jack-ma-covid-19.

216 Ouma, Polet Njeri, Abednego Nzyuko Masai, and Israel Nyaburi Nyadera, "Health coverage and what Kenya can learn from the COVID-19 pandemic," *Journal of Global Health*, vol. 10, No. 2 (2020), doi: 10.7189/jogh.10.020362.

test kits, therapeutics and vaccines, arises from the newly-minted 'COVID millionaires.'

KEMSA Procurement and COVID 'Millionaires'

'COVID millionaires' quickly became a moniker for the procurement corruption scandal that rocked the Kenya Medical Supplies Agency (KEMSA). It also refers to the process through which companies that were registered within a day won anywhere from millions to billions of shillings in contracts to supply PPE. The contracts were awarded in highly dubious procurement circumstances, although in emergencies, government agencies have some leeway to waive the procurement standards. The 'successful' 'contractors' were supposed to supply the government and designated hospitals and institutions with PPE. Overall, 'COVID millionaires' involved vast sums of money, starting with a US$2 billion (Kshs. 200 billion) mix of aid and grants to fight the pandemic.[217]

In the first instance, Kshs. 780 million that was intended for PPE for healthcare workers and hospitals was misappropriated and the PPE, if at all procured, did not reach those that were at the frontlines of a rapidly spreading and barely contained pandemic. When they did, some of the PPE supplied was deemed quite unsatisfactory. An audit found "substandard gloves, hazmat suits and faceshields,"[218] while hazard pay as a result of working in such high-risk environments was not forthcoming. These low—quality supplies were estimated to cause, directly or indirectly, 10 deaths among doctors and medical practitioners. An example of the egregiousness of the 'COVID millionaires' was the case of 'Shop and Buy Ltd.,' which was formed and within weeks, won a Kshs. 1 billion tender illustrate the brazenness of the COVID millionaires.[219]

Some of the companies formed to bid for the COVID-19 funds were also suspected of being connected to politicians. But squarely in the sights of the allegations was the head of KEMSA, Jonah Manjari, who oscillated his defense between 'instructions from above' to 'no money was lost', to 'orders from the Cabinet Secretary and the Permanent Secretary' to other more far-fetched explanations. What became clear was that there was a stink, and while

---

[217] Emmanuel Igunza, "Coronavirus corruption in Kenya: Officials and businesspeople targeted," *BBC News*, Nairobi, 24 September 2020, https://www.bbc.com/news/world-africa-54278417.

[218] Igunza, "Coronavirus corruption in Kenya," (2020).

[219] Igunza, "Coronavirus corruption in Kenya," (2020).

the government has pledged to keep investigating, it is clear that even this will go the way of the NYS, Anglo Leasing or Goldenberg scandals. After taking quite a bit of heat from the public, the beneficiaries of the KEMSA debacle, the Public Procurement Information Portal (PPIP) published the names of the beneficiaries (companies).

However, because the Ethics and Anti-Corruption Commission (EACC) took over the investigative matter into potential fraud, freezing all payments, KEMSA and its suppliers "are caught in a dilemma on how to deal with the losses from the Sh. 6.2 billion stock stuck at its warehouses, some of which is expiring."[220] The entire situation then became tragically ironic: on the one hand, the 'sh. 6.2 billion stock stuck at its warehouses' is needed now, not in future, to help fight especially the spiking COVID-19 (delta variant) infections. On the other, it was almost as predictable as sunrise, that there would be a scandal around KEMSA and PPE procurement. The EACC "froze all payments to the companies" pending investigations, to "stop another Sh. 9 billion that was to be paid out."[221] Given the perishable nature of some of the goods, and the murkiness of who foots bill for purchased supplies, this risks to further imperil the country, and make recovery from COVID-19 even more difficult.

An optimist might believe that the investigations will someday, perhaps even soon, produce results and the culprits who misappropriated PPE found and prosecuted. However, if Goldenberg, NYS, Anglo-Leasing, police communications equipment, Kenya's Embassy in Tokyo, the Naval Ship procurement and other numerous 'financially suspect events' are any indicators, one would do well to focus on using leaves from the blue gum tree and '*Wanjirũ wa rurii*' as potential therapeutics, even possible cures for COVID-19 than the prospect of unearthing the who, what, where, when and how of the COVID-19 funds, or more broadly, how a government keeps losing money to corruption, to 'cabals' that the health CS had vowed to fight and which seem to have drawn him into their hydra-headed graft.

There is a final element of potential 'institutional graft' that may further imperil the fight against COVID-19. Although this is mostly hearsay, speculation is rife, that Kenya pretends to have more COVID-19 cases than it actually has. This is almost believable, if one examines citizens' behavior, in order to attract more funding so that the *wenye-nchi* can continue benefitting

---

[220] Paul Wafula, "At long last, faces of Covid-19 millionaires start emerging," *Nation Media Group*, Tuesday, November 24, 2020, https://nation.africa/kenya/news/at-long-last-faces-of-covid-19-millionaires-start-emerging--3208076?view=htmlamp.

[221] Wafula, "At long last, faces of COVID-10 millionaires," (2020), n.p.

from foreign assistance provided to fight the pandemic. This is the pernicious nature of corruption. Even worse, it does, rather predictably, enhance the lack of trust in 'institutions of government.' The latter is a most troubling turn, one that is not easily remedied. For even when the political process changes the nation's leader (president) and the executive – e.g., Cabinet Secretaries or other high-level functionaries, it still retains those other structures that citizens interact with most, such as police officers and chiefs. It is not clear how this problem might be solved. What is undeniable is that COVID-19's spread is benefitting from a government and citizenry that suffer from a permanent paralysis in tackling corruption.

Economic Slowdowns, Shutdowns and Government Responses

Responses to the COVID-19 pandemic across the world shared some across-the-board elements, the most important being public health, epidemiological, administrative, and socio-economic responses. In the latter, countries differed in terms of the extent to which they addressed these issues, the support they provided (if any), and the length of time through which they provided (or not) such support and the impact such assistance had on citizens. Most initial research regarding the COVID-19 pandemic year(s) has shown an overwhelmingly negative impacts of the COVID-19 pandemic across several measures. Salient examples of these impacts include 55.6% 'vulnerably employed' workers in Pakistan,[222] 39.1 percent fall in Rwanda's GDP for 2020,[223] and 75.8 percent decline in work in the food services sector over a 5-week lockdown period in Africa's largest economy, Nigeria.[224]

Kenyans were in dire straits, as shown by FAO's data on prevalence of undernourishment and further evidenced by the 2020 Global Hunger Index. As of 2016, almost 10 million Kenyans were undernourished, accounting for 21.1% of the population.[225] The country has seen a gradual decrease in the

---

[222] Muhammad Saad Moeen, Zeeshan Haider, Sania Haider Shikoh, Noormah Rizwan, Stephen Davies and Abdul Wajid Rana, *COVID-19: Estimating impact on the economy and poverty in Pakistan: Using the SAM Multiplier Model*, (Pakistan: IFPRI/PACE, 2020).

[223] Emerta Aragie, Xinshen Diao, Sherman Robinson, Gracie Rosenbach, David J. Spielman, and James Thurlow, *Assessing the economy-wide impacts of COVID-19 on Rwanda's economy, agri-food system, and poverty*, Strategy Support Program/Working Paper 01, (Kigali, Rwanda: IFPRI Rwanda, 2021).

[224] Andam, Kwaw S. Andam, Hyacinth Edeh, Victor Oboh, Karl Pauw, and James Thurlow, *Estimating the economic costs of COVID-19 in Nigeria*, (Lagos: IFPRI Nigeria, 2020).

[225] FAO, IFAD and WFP, *The State of Food Insecurity in the World 2015, Meeting the 2015 international hunger targets: taking stock of uneven progress*, (Rome: FAO, 2015).

percentage of undernourished Kenyans (from a high of 32.4% in 1990-1992), the 12% drop over 20 years has likely been reversed by the pandemic. This is borne by 2020 fata, ranking Kenya 85th (out of 107 countries') with a serious (23.7) level of hunger.[226] The proportion of undernourished population tracks with the FAO data. Prevalence of stunting in children less than five years old has decreased from a high of 40% in 200 to 31% in 2020. This does not even take into account the conditions being experienced by refugees, of whom Kenya hosts a substantial number in refugee camps in the north of the country.[227]

Country-level data sheds more light on how Kenya's government's lack of robust food assistance program even during the pandemic has undermined the fight to contain the pandemic, by giving citizens (dis)-incentive to flout COVID-19 guidelines, facing the choice between starvation or contracting the virus. Even the well-meaning face these kinds of dilemmas of common aversions: avoid COVID-19 and starvation. But absent government assistance, one has no choice but to find some means of sustenance. Kenya's early data mirrors that of other African countries, ranging from the deleterious impact on the 83.6% of Kenyan workers who are employed in the informal sector and for whom the incremental COVID-19 mitigation strategies such as lockdowns, cessation of movement and increases in the prices of basic commodities and transportation costs as a result of social-distancing increases citizens' costs without corresponding governmental aid.[228]

That said, there was a recognition that mandating a shut-down *and* not providing a mitigation strategy towards the hunger that was inevitable (and already existing before COVID-19) was a thoroughly self-defeating strategy, which led to the policy actions aimed at addressing income loss and broader social support for the citizenry. One of the earliest actions was the announcement, on March 25th, of Kshs. 10 billion (US$100 million) to supplement the fund for the elderly, orphans and the medically 'compromised,' although it is not clear that there are active, reasonable, manipulation-free and fool-proof criteria for these determinations.

---

[226] Global Hunger Index, "Kenya," *Global Hunger Index*, 2020, https://www.globalhungerindex.org/kenya.html.

[227] IOM & WFP, "Populations at risk: Implications of COVID-19 for hunger, migration and displacement: An Analysis of Food Security Trends in Major Migration Hotspots," *World Food Programme (WFP) and the International Organization for Migration* (IOM), November 2020, https://www.iom.int/sites/default/files/populations_at_risk_-_implications_of_covid-19_for_hunger_migration_and_displacement.pdf.

[228] Maureen Were, "COVID-19 and socioeconomic impact in Africa: The case of Kenya," *UNU-WIDER, WIDER Background Note* | 3/2020 (Helsinki: UNU-WIDER, 2020).

As part of the mitigation strategies, the president outlined an "8-Point Economic Stimulus Programme, amounting to a total of Kshs. 53.7 billion."[229] The government pledged Kshs. 250 million a month to be distributed to 'vulnerable families.' Estimates suggest that near 18 million Kenyans (35%) live in poverty, at or below the US$1.90 a day. The Kshs. 250 million a month in food assistance that the government pledged thus amounts to less than a pittance: an average of Kshs. 13.89 per person. A 400-gram loaf of bread costs about Kshs. 50.

It is not quite clear what this might purchase, particularly for an entire month, considering then that any of the members of these families can only spend Kshs. 0.46 a day. Were the government to use the World Bank's poverty lines, Kshs. 3,352 (rural areas) and Kshs. 5,995 (urban areas) per person (adult equivalent terms) for both food and non-food items, and assuming a 50% urbanization (poverty) rate, the government would spend Kshs. 30 billion a month on the 9 million 'vulnerable' rural persons alone, and almost double that amount for the urban 'vulnerable.' Clearly, the amount that the government pledged to spend is nowhere close to that amount, or sufficient, and one wonders about the utility of the so-called government assistance. One surmises that being seen to do something, rather than actually doing something that makes a difference, was the essence of the impact.

The distribution of the Pandemic Cash Transfer Program has also been dubious in both its goals and implementation. HRW analysis of government data concluded that "the Covid-19 cash transfer program provided support to less than five percent of the socio-economically vulnerable families in Nairobi" and thus "failed to guarantee the right to an adequate standard of living for more than 95 percent of vulnerable households."[230] Even the president admitted to the challenges of attempting to distribute food, noting that "half the financial resources given to relief suppliers were LOST to BROKERS and logistics"[231] (original emphasis). Even in a pandemic, it was clear that self-interest trumped any consideration of fair distribution of food, while logistics have become a delaying tactic and source of funds' diversion for private use.

---

[229] PSCU, "The Seventh Presidential Address on the Coronavirus Pandemic," (2020), n.p.

[230] HRW, 'We Are All Vulnerable Here': Kenya's Pandemic Cash Transfer Program Riddled With Irregularities," *Human Rights Watch,* July 20th, 2021, https://www.hrw.org/report/2021/07/20/we-are-all-vulnerable-here/kenyas-pandemic-cash-transfer-program-riddled.

[231] PSCU, "The Seventh Presidential Address on the Coronavirus Pandemic," (2020), n.p.

The formula for the distribution of the cash was also unspecified and therefore subject to some manipulation. For instance, if one were to focus on those who lost jobs in the formal sector, the number would only account for about 17% of the population. Conversely, if the government were to assume that everyone with a 'job' could qualify for the assistance, and near 83% of the population works in the informal sector, it would be a challenge to decide whether even farmers would qualify under this 'informal sector' designation, or if the classification only extends to the '*jua kali*' sector. Thus, providing assistance to all citizens who wanted it would have been more prudent. As part of economic measures, the government engaged 26,000 youths with a pledge to increase the number to 200,000, "engaging them in the National Hygiene Programme – Kazi Mtaani Initiative,"[232] at a cost of Kshs. 10 billion.

Regarding the actual 'economic stimulus measures,' the president's speech highlighted 8 points which were quite diverse, but based on work, rather than simply giving cash assistance. Infrastructure rehabilitation, at a cost of Kshs. 5 billion of local labor would be the first item on the agenda. Others included education (the phased re-opening of schools), with Kshs. 6.5 billion set aside to hire 10,000 teachers, 1,000 ICT interns and to support local artisans by procuring 250,000 locally-made desks. Notably, there was not significant investment in ICT educational content delivery, Wi-Fi or the related peripherals, or mention of the now abortive School Laptop Project. The third of the 8-point program targeted SMEs, at an allocation of Kshs. 13 billion; 10 billion for VAT refunds and Kshs. 3 billion as SME credit guarantee scheme for micro-enterprises. A further allocation of Kshs. 30 billion was set aside to pay balances in the road construction sector, which was especially vibrant.[233]

The fourth area was slated to be health, with a proposed increase in the number of healthcare workers by 5,000 to serve for a year, in part to fight COVID-19 and to work towards meeting the goal of Universal Health Coverage (UHC), increasing research capacity in medical facilities and improve performance, as well as use Kshs. 1.7 billion to increase the bed capacity, using *Jua Kali* sector expertise. Agriculture was the fifth sector, with Kshs. 3 billion earmarked for farm inputs purchase for 200,000 small scale farmers (another pittance, considering almost 60 percent of Kenya's population, almost 20 million, is involved in farming). Horticulture would benefit from Kshs. 1.5 billion including to access international markets,

[232] PSCU, "The Seventh Presidential Address on the Coronavirus Pandemic," (2020), n.p.
[233] PSCU, "The Seventh Presidential Address on the Coronavirus Pandemic," (2020), n.p.

although the ban on flights would be a major hindrance in accomplishing this goal, together with the changed spending habits by most horticultural product consumers especially in Europe and North America.

Tourism, the sixth sector and traditionally one of the country's more robust foreign exchange earners – and therefore, a major employer – also suffered significant setbacks. They varied: some were as a result of movement restrictions within the country, or lockdowns. Others were external but had implications for Kenya, such as foreign countries and the major sources of tourists, imposing quarantine requirements on returning citizens and residents. This thoroughly discouraged foreign travel, but the unpredictable nature of the pandemic, lack of a vaccine and general uncertainty was a contributor to decreasing tourism. The sector was set to benefit from Kshs. 2 billion, and soft loans were to be provided through the Tourism Finance Corporation (TFC). The program proposed to ensure that there would be post-pandemic supply of trained industry professionals.

Environmental concerns constituted the seventh element of the president's plan. In it, Kenyatta articulated the government's objective of rehabilitating select infrastructure including water wells, water storage and transmission facilities, and a renewed focus on ASAL areas, flood control and general environmental activities under the 'Greening Kenya Campaign.' These initiatives were projected to cost Kshs. 2.3 billion. The eighth point was in manufacturing, including spending Kshs. 600 to purchase locally manufactured vehicles. This provided some impetus to build – 'Buy Kenya Build Kenya' campaign,[234] help sustain local manufacturing and industry, but more importantly, to 'deficit-spend' and support Kenyans through business and employment.

Educational Responses and Impacts

Just as the business world was unprepared for the pandemic, it was immediately abundantly clear that the Kenyan educational system was just not built to operate at distance, online, virtually, or in a pandemic. It became clear too, that despite the occasional tinkering with the system, there was not much change and the desired skills to change the nation into an exports manufacturer was not going as intended. Still the colonial-era, highly racist and discriminatory 7-4-2-3 3-in-1 system with different facilities, schools and

---

[234] PSCU, "The Seventh Presidential Address on the Coronavirus Pandemic," (2020), n.p.

experiences for Asian, African and European students apparently fostered elitist, individualistic attitudes. It was also accused of failing to equip learners with practical skills compatible with Kenya's post-independence needs. As such, the 'reformist' 8-4-4 was geared towards equipping learners with practical skills and (a tad suspicious version of) patriotism, while the new CBC is intended to decrease emphasis on exams and foster students' interests and abilities, turning them into careers. Still, the current, two-track (CBC and 8-4-4) system is hardly built for the early 20th century, as the pandemic made clear.

Notwithstanding what name or educational system is in use, what passes for most schools is i) buildings, ii) teachers, iii) wooden desks (where available) or long, wooden benches with kids packed like sardines next to each other. For play and equipment, there is mostly grassy spaces masquerading as playing fields even in slums, destined to produce international soccer stars (such as Denis Oliech) and world class athletes such as Faith Kipyegon. For school-grown athletic talent, by some magic, Kenya has continued to dominate, perhaps because some students must undertake a marathon each morning to get to school and each evening to get home before total darkness; and repeat next day. Some school buildings are trees, some are adobe, mud-walled enterprises. Some get swept away every time there is a flood, and some never get rebuilt. Private schools often have better facilities and resources, but they are fewer and have far fewer students. They often cater to the well-off.

But, with remarkable foresight, even the shacks benefitted from the government's school electrification project, which saw all public primary schools connected to the electrical grid between 2014 and 2016, so that by the end of 2016, all 23,375 public primary schools, and 9,431 public secondary schools were connected.[235] However, that left yet another challenge: few schools have the set-up, knowhow or capacity to deliver content from distance, not just because they do not have the equipment, but also because of training, storage, electrical supply (electrification is *not* the same as supplying electric power). And despite the notion that the 8-4-4 education system would equip the learners with practical skills to navigate even these challenges (think solar power), there is not much evidence that this has been accomplished.

---

[235] The World Bank, "Kenya National Electrification Strategy: Key Highlights," The World Bank Group, 2018, https://pubdocs.worldbank.org/en/413001554284496731/Kenya-National-Electrification-Strategy-KNES-Key-Highlights-2018.pdf.

School Is More Than Learning: School Nutrition

More importantly, considering the levels of poverty that pervade Kenya, few students would have the resources (internet-capable smart phones, computers, laptops *in their homes* or the time when out of school, to enable access to such (any) online content. And we haven't even started addressing the issue of internet connectivity, bundles and costs, which are estimated to be some of the highest in Africa. Not unique to Africa, the pandemic and move to online teaching also exposed the gap that is growing between educators and learners: while the latter have an increasing grasp of technology and use of devices, the same cannot be said for the potential content creators and deliverers, i.e., the teachers and professors. This is true in Kenya. Thus, even as UNESCO was estimating that 98% of all 1.8 billion students across the world were affected by COVID-19, for some it was more impactful.[236]

School closures often affected pupils and students in rural areas more than contemporaries in urban areas. Rural students (almost 85 percent of all enrolled students) were already facing major inequalities in educational access and resources. Specialty programs are few and far between, and as such, learners with disabilities, pupils and students in slums, refugee camps, IDP camps and informal settlements, farthest reaches of the country and those whose parents lost income due to the restrictions would have been especially (if they are not) disadvantaged. Some of the said learners often come from nomadic communities who may not place a high value on education, and as such, any reason to *not* educate especially the girl child becomes an opportunity to save money and probably make more money by marrying them off. It is hardly conceivable that these communities living in such – including nomadic environments – would afford to acquire the necessary, online learning resources such as computers, software and other peripherals, financially and psychologically, or have the competency to use them as intended.[237]

There were other even more significant issues with the suspension of in-school learning, for both primary and secondary schools. For pupils who attend school in Arid and Semi-Arid Lands (ASALs) in Kenya – which encompasses 29 of 47 counties covering 80% of Kenya's lands, school also

---

[236] Areba George Ngwacho, "COVID-19 Pandemic Impact on Kenyan Education Sector: Learner Challenges and Mitigations," *Journal of Research Innovation and Implications in Education*, Vol. 4, No. 2 (2020), 128-139, https://jriiejournal.com/wp-content/uploads/2021/03/JRIIE-4-2-015.pdf.

[237] Ngwacho, "COVID-19 Pandemic Impact on Kenyan Education Sector," (2020).

offers opportunity for more than education: nutrition.[238] The impact of school closure was wider than just the students themselves: it "ended school meals, which used to provide considerable market opportunity for local food producers and traders,"[239] thus further impacting local economies and communities. For urban areas, this was even more impactful, taken together with the restrictions and scale-backs in in-person business activities, where some (many) low-income residents depend on physically being at work to make money often on a daily basis. The net effect will include an increase in undernourishment (which stood at 29.4% of total population, 2016-8) and anemia (27.2% in 2016).[240] Both of these conditions mostly affect school-going children.

News reports have also regularly highlighted other deleterious impacts of COVID-19 and the closure of learning institutions. These reported cases have included violence against children, early marriages, FGM and an increase in the number of reported rapes, including of minors, sometimes by their very caregivers. As such, the safety of schools, even absent 'mandated reporting,' makes the vulnerable children even more likely to face abuse. The possibility of many students regressing, failing to retain learnt content, experiencing significant gaps between school terms and even forgetting the materials learnt, even though they would face exams in rapid succession in order to keep the calendar on schedule, has to be taken into account. Some students have stayed out of school for almost six months at different times, and it is not clear that this is conducive to performance.

A complete revisit and analysis of the ways in which education in Kenya has been impacted by COVID-19 would be superfluous, especially considering the systematic way that other researchers have addressed this particular issue. According to Ngwacho, COVID-19 brought about an increase in the physical distance between students and pupils with their teachers due to social distancing), even though this distance wasn't narrowed by virtual contact. Secondly, although public libraries are not quite as widely spread as in the west, both school and public libraries became inaccessible, robbing pupils and students an additional source of learning. A third outcome relates to the financing of school fees and other related charges when schools finally

---

[238] IUCN, "Kenya - Arid and semi-arid lands," *International Union for Conservation of Nature (IUCN),* 2021, https://www.iucn.org/restoration-initiative/projects/kenya-arid-and-semi-arid-lands.

[239] Mulat Demeke, Josphat Kariuki and Mercy Wanjiru, "Assessing the Impact of COVID-19 on Food and Nutrition Security and Adequacy of Responses in Kenya," *Food and Agriculture Organization of the United Nations*, Policy Brief, May 2020.

[240] Demeke, et al. "Assessing the Impact of COVID-19 on Food and Nutrition," (2020).

resumed, due to job and income loss. Paying for the required supplies such as meals, books and other learning materials especially within the CBC curriculum became even more difficult and further set some students back.[241]

Uncommon Impacts of Interrupted Learning

Sexual and Gender Based Violence (SGBV), while a perennial societal – and Kenyan – issue, has been especially magnified by the pandemic. Both in Kenya and in other countries, schools serve additional functions, including being safe havens, or 'social protection hubs,' against social ills such as SGBV, according to Ngwacho. With school closures, home-schooling is an exceedingly difficult proposition for most Kenyans, but social protections are also lost, leading to the widespread reports of violence, rape and other abuses in the home. For girls from certain parts of the country where early marriages are prevalent, FGM is widely practiced and girl child education less favored, the loss of support and programming that often keeps them from these outcomes magnified the peril they faced.

But more broadly, and with regard to sexual offences, recent data has shown "that child victims are younger, more likely to be victimized by a neighbor in a private residence, and in the daytime, compared to pre-pandemic."[242] Relatives and care-givers have also increasingly become accused of perpetrating these crimes, and school-age children have fewer reporting avenues during the pandemic. Boekart, et al. find that in Kenya, "SGBV cases had tripled in the first three months of the dusk-to-dawn curfew and the national GBV hotline, in June 2020, reported a 650% increase in calls since the implementation of the COVID-19 mitigation measures."[243]

There was also a significant uptick in reports of teenage pregnancies and therewith, abortions, some that were performed under inherently unsafe conditions. Considering UNFPA's estimate of "31 million additional SGBV

---

[241] Ngwacho, "COVID-19 Pandemic Impact on Kenyan Education Sector," (2020), 132.

[242] Laura M. Stevens, James C. Rockey, Sarah R. Rockowitz, Wangu Kanja, Melissa F. Colloff and Heather D. Flowe, "Children's Vulnerability to Sexual Violence During COVID-19 in Kenya: Recommendations for the Future," *Frontiers in Global Women's Health*, Vol. 2, (2021), 1-5, https://doi.org/10.3389/fgwh.2021.630901.

[243] Clara Broekaert, Ceri-Lune Renneboog, Ferdinand Okwaro, Abdu Mohiddin, and Marleen Temmerman, "Working Paper - Digital News Media Coverage on Sexual and Gender-based Violence in Kenya: Scoping the Impact of the COVID-19 Pandemic," *SocArXiv*, (Jan. 10, 2021). doi:10.31235/osf.io/vbku6.

cases worldwide,"[244] after six months of lockdown (now more than a year and a half), the issue has been especially pertinent, particularly given that the Kenyan society is loath to address reproductive health consistently. The flip-side to the negative impacts of the school closures due to COVID-19 is pupils and students' own conduct: there was reported an increase in 'behavioral issues' among learners, perhaps understandable given the heightened distress. But some of it arises from the practicalities of decentralized structure and authority that is home. Working parents cannot always supervise learners, and when left alone, the already-stressed (working) parents have to deal with substance abuse, rebelliousness and other truancy.

In addition, due to the conditions of many homes, access to audio, visual and digital content was uneven, even non-existent especially in homes that are quite basic (e.g., adobe, thatched houses). Despite the Ministry of Education's 2018 attempt at crafting emergency and disaster management contingency plans for education, the actual implementation was still under consideration. While ICT is not necessarily directly related to disaster management, and ought to *also* be implemented during other times, the pandemic is arguably a disaster that *required* ICT infrastructure to be in place or be rapidly deployable and with enough trained personnel to carry out the necessary instruction, repair, maintenance, and especially importantly, content creation.

Even where ICT use was possible, numerous constraints did, and still do exist, to challenge any such possibilities. Notably, "a survey by ICT Authority revealed that MoE has not installed CBC content into digital devices 3 years since its inception."[245] The hype of the school laptop project that was highly touted before the 2013 general election has remained a fading mirage. In itself, the proposal to provide first grade learners with laptops was especially ill-conceived. It may have been merely a campaign promise, but the 12-year gap between first grade ICT users' first use, and their graduation from high school more than a decade later, ignored the rapid pace of technological developments, UNESCO's proposal that early schooling years be conducted in learners' own first language (mother tongues – of which there is not enough, if any electronic content), and the lack of training of teachers.

With regard to the discussion on the pandemic's nutritional impacts, there was an increase in hunger among children especially in the ASAL regions. Absent strategies or mechanisms to distribute food to the pupils or the homes of otherwise eligible pupils and students, and the inaccessibility of homes in

---

[244] Stevens, et al., "Children's Vulnerability to Sexual Violence during COVID-19 in Kenya," (2021), n.p.

[245] Ngwacho, "COVID-19 Pandemic Impact on Kenyan Education Sector," (2020), 133.

slums, ASAL areas and clashes-prone regions, nutrition has suffered. With 29 of the 47 of the country's counties classified as ASAL, and the simultaneous locust invasion that begun late in 2019, and which has continued to occur in waves, devastating crops, reducing harvests and imperiling any food security that might have been achieved especially in the region,[246]one expects that school-going children are further, and importantly, negatively affected. Future studies will likely shed more light on the overall long-term COVID-19 outcomes on nutrition.

Majority of Kenya's current educational system is overwhelmingly based on exams. It is a most untenable proposition that is addressed by the Competency-Based Curriculum (CBC). CBC is in the process of being implemented; thus, some students have to focus on national exams through KCPE and KCSE, the quintessential pathways to perceived future through academic achievement. The numbers are dire: of the approximate 1 million pupils that join standard (grade) 1, approximately 100,000 (or 10%) 'pass' to join university, implying the country has an educational system that produces '90% failures.' Besides the irony of an *education* system doing that, the pressure on students as exams approach is one of the most significant student stressors. The shortened school term without necessarily varying the exams has put immense pressure on learners, parents and teachers alike: to perform well, to teach the same materials in an abridged school term, and to find resources to support learners respectively.

Government policy and the education CS' pronouncements have generally done little, if anything to alleviate anxiety around examinations and performance, even from the very beginning of the pandemic. As an example, in managing the education sector as COVID-19 cases started going up in early 2020, the CS "indicated that Kenyan schools will remain closed for the next one month [...] the CS, however, reported that the national examinations for primary and secondary schools remain on schedule."[247] The heightened pressure on students increased behavioral issues and anxiety, which is felt even more by students from disadvantaged homes, for they often lack the resources to learn from home, which explains some of the successes of the boarding school: fewer distractions. In normal circumstances, students with marginal means would already be facing steep odds given resource constraints and some environments that are less conducive for studying.

---

[246] Sharmila Devi, "Locust swarms in East Africa could be 'a catastrophe,'" *The Lancet*, Vol 395 (February 22, 2020), p. 542. doi: https://doi.org/10.1016/S0140-6736(20)30406-2 add this to the references for section.

[247] Ngwacho, "COVID-19 Pandemic Impact on Kenyan Education Sector," (2020), 133.

There was an additional, related issue that further increased the challenges to parents: finding the means to pay for their children's tuition, in a pandemic with job and business losses. A recalibrated educational calendar, necessary given closures to contain the pandemic and the need to retool schools to conform to COVID-19 mitigation measures, meant shorter school terms, without any corresponding or significant reduction in school fees or other form of government assistance. It is also useful to recall that most parents are farmers (accounting for about 60% of economic activity), and use their farm proceeds to pay school fees. Short-term crops do grow inside 3-4 months, maize and other cash crops up to 9 months. A 2-month school term with a 1-week break induces stress: crops are not going to grow any faster just because there is a pandemic and school terms have been shortened.

Specifically, from the education ministry's published guidelines, the school year began on July 27th, 2020. The calendar requires students to learn for 2 months (not the usual 3), close for a week and resume the 2nd term in October, close in December for a week, and reopen for the 3rd term in January, concluding that school year in March 2022. A normal school year is usually 9 months long; this version will only be 6 months. Pressure for all stakeholders to excel in their relative tasks under these circumstances often sits more harshly on parents' shoulders. Stress on parents can lead to negative outcomes, including inability to pay for the schooling and therefore, increased school dropouts, distress in homes, or parental (frustration) violence to be directed at children.

Discrimination against those who have been infected with the COVID-19 virus has been rife despite everyone having lungs. Phrases such as 'yule wa COVID' are prevalent, and in no way discriminate. Although COVID-19 has been around for over 600 days, the stigma has not lessened. The fact that its effects on children who might catch the virus have so far been more mild (at least considering the first few variants), the stigma has regularly extended to learners. Given the absence of counseling services in schools, it is not clear what such labels might do to such students even after schools resumed. But it is also not clear that schools are practicing mitigation measures, especially social distancing, given the usual crowding in schools. One cannot argue that new schools were built so as to facilitate physical separation, and so the virus continues to circulate even amongst pupils and therefore to their families. And if the rest of the country provides any insight, there is no expectation of better use of masks among pupils than there is among the general public.[248]

---

[248] Ngwacho, "COVID-19 Pandemic Impact on Kenyan Education Sector," (2020), 134.

A final impact of the pandemic on the educational system is less academic and related to developing the 'whole person'; academically, physically and recreationally. Co– or extra–curricular activities are a major feature of the secondary school education level. Because of the pandemic's transmission pathways, few schools now offer opportunities for students to participate in these activities, including sports, games, clubs, music and drama festivals. Non-participation diminishes the available opportunities for socialization within and between schools and among students.

The interruption in the non-curricular activities also inhibits potential development of other skills that may have undergirded the foundation of Lupita Nyong'o's Hollywood career. It is the case that most learners are directed to and encouraged to excel academically, but there are other pathways to socio-economic success in future, through these creative and performative endeavors. Participation in these activities also regularizes an otherwise elitist education system with too much focus on academic achievement, potentially decreasing chances for students to discover other, potential career pathways. British-Nigerian comedian Gina Yashere may have said it in jest, but most African parents direct their kids to four (five) careers, i.e., "doctor, lawyer, engineer, accountant and disgrace to the family."[249]

Pandemic Blues and a More Equitable Kenya

The foregoing has illuminated some of the challenges that Kenya has faced as a result of the COVID-19 pandemic, over the past two years. While it is admirable that the country did not shut down educational institutions so as to deal with the pandemic, we still have to recognize that educational achievement has been negatively impacted, particularly as the country was transitioning to a new educational system. It is necessary to learn from the lessons of the past - after all, that is what has moved humanity forward - and fireproof the country for the next pandemic. In the education sector, the pandemic exposed the realities that Kenyan education has not changed for a century. The closure of educational institutions illuminated the technology gap, even as we live in the information age. It is necessary to ensure that

[249] LSSC, "Gina Yashere Built Elevators before Becoming a Comedian," The Late Show with Stephen Colbert, March 20, 2021, https://web.facebook.com/colbertlateshow/videos/482624979775308/.

students' learning, the development of the future human resource the country will depend on, is uninterrupted.

In terms of corruption, it would be akin to beating a dead horse, to keep reiterating what has been obvious since the country's founding. Corruption has been with Kenya as much as its national anthem or flag. it is a vice the government and society have been unable to eradicate. It touches on every aspect of life, and there is great temptation to give up on ever fixing it. As such, it would have been anomalous, if especially the World Bank COVID-19 funding, and perhaps too, China's PPE and food assistance during the pandemic, had not been misappropriated and misspent. The idea that we hurt ourselves and our countrymen has never seemed to resonate or change behavior in the procurement processes in our institutions, or the inability to prosecute graft. One can only assume that the prosecutors must have a vested interest in not prosecuting. But, it bodes poorly for the ability to manage the pandemic. There is perhaps no better explanation of how we do this, than the idea of cutting off one's nose to spite their face.

COVID-19 has also exposed other weaknesses within the economy and societal processes. Kenya has a very limited welfare system, which seems to only address the concerns of the elderly and infirm, and even then, only a select 240,000 out of 1.9 million aged 65 and over. The broader absence of a social safety net was exposed as a concern: when the government shut down many firms that specialize in face-to-face business, and imposed curfews, which impacted the ability to sell farm produce, milk and other similar products, the levels of income went down. Unsubsidized, Kenyans faced a most between-the-devil-and-the-deep-blue-sea situation: catch COVID-19 while working to feed the family, or starve with the family but comply with government regulations. The way the country deals with division of labor is also important, because women have seemed to bear the greatest burden for the provision of daily sustenance, while also taking care of those who caught COVID-19. The inequity and suspect government policy exposed in these COVID-19 times deserves reconsideration.

Chapter 6

Socio-Cultural Traditions, Religious Observances and Community Responses

Abstract

This chapter addresses some of the most pernicious issues that have impacted COVID-19 responses in Kenya, namely, issues associated with the widely-practised socio-cultural traditions, practices and religious beliefs. Kenya is a motley collection of 43+ ethnic groups, with a variety but significant number of traditional practices by each, such as circumcision, bride-wealth and dowry payment, marriage ceremonies, burial ceremonies and other cultural festivals. Most of these are accompanied by festivals with singing, dancing and close contact, the very essence of the COVID-19 transmission pathways. Being a critical part of the identity and belief, societies are loathe to give up, or even modify their conduct. Likewise, while most Kenyans profess the Christian faith (about 80%), there are significant Muslim, Hindu and African Traditional Religion adherents. All these religions come with religious observances and ceremonies such as baptism, naming, 'reception' into the congregation, burial and even basic religious services. Further, the communitarian nature of African societies sees a lot of *harambees,* in-person versions of GoFundMe to cover all manner of financial deficits within communities and families; these too would be affected by lockdowns. Like many other countries, these were the first to be stopped, essentially banned. Unlike other countries, conducting them online was a significant challenge. The implementation of the social-distancing and outlawing of the socio-cultural and traditional activities indeed set the government up against some of the most powerful congregations and groups. Coupled with the elites' behaviors of political rallies – and even simple activities such as super-markets, which saw many groups of people essentially congregating, they set up areas of conflict with the government. These conflicts and the accommodations are outlined in this chapter.

A Complex, Religious Nation: Religious Responses

Politics and faith are some of the most significant areas of peoples' lives, but occasionally, also the most pertinent sources of societal strife. The foundations of both are largely inexplicable, sometimes defy logic, but are critical elements of most peoples' being, especially religion. Political and faith forums, however, served as some of the most contested spaces as far as managing COVID—19 is concerned. Across the world, political positions have influenced even simple public health responses, including, for example, whether to wear a mask or not. In Kenya, the fervent belief in one's political position relative to the concurrent BBI initiative that was gaining steam and collecting signatures pre-empted the possibility of ending political activities. Given that the appellate courts ultimately scuttled the BBI process, it is regrettable that the process of campaigning for BBI, and of collecting requisite signatures, may have led to some infections.

But more importantly, as social beings that regularly appeal to African traditions alongside religion, these became even more contested than the political spaces. Add this to the reality of different religious beliefs, three major religions in the country (not counting the traditional and less mainstream religious such as Rastafarians or African Traditional Religions), and the church's position on vaccines and worship, religious services and events became both a flashpoint over closures but also possible COVID-19 incubators. The unrestrained political activity that continued, in light of popularization of the BBI initiative, cast a light on the perceived hypocrisy of calls for suspension of religious activities – and with good reason. Add these two major incidents to the overall skepticism that COVID-19 existed in the first place, and the ingredients for a perfect pandemic storm were in place.

Religious services, especially churches and particularly with examples from North America, South Korea and across Africa, have already been shown to be COVID-19 'superspreader' events. But even before the more recent outbreaks, it was already clear that religious communities were some of the incubators of the virus. A study published in 2021 found high seroprevalence rates amongst 'geographically distinct yet culturally bound religious [Jewish] communities'[250] across the US, rising to a 32.5% in New Jersey; this was long

[250] Israel Zyskind, Avi Z. Rosenberg, Jason Zimmerman, Hiam Naiditch, Aaron E. Glatt, Abraham Pinter, Elitza S. Theel, Michael J. Joyner, D. Ashley Hill, Miriam R. Lieberman, Elliot Bigajer, Daniel Stok, Elliot Frank and Jonathan I. Silverberg, "SARS-CoV-2 Seroprevalence and Symptom Onset in Culturally Linked Orthodox Jewish Communities

before other outbreaks in South Korea and elsewhere. The world would soon come to recognize both the challenges inherent in curtailing religious (and political) meets even in the name of public health, to the extent that it would need to appeal to the highest religious authorities of *all* faiths, to provide impetus to conform to the limitations and even accept vaccines.

Although Kenya's government articulated containment measures as early as 20th March, 2020, with in-person religious services suspended as early as March 29th, religious figures were already, and in time, going to take cues from religious leaders and others who downplayed the potential impact of COVID-19. To wit, "Tanzania President John Magufuli has said COVID-19 is the work of the devil and public worship in churches and mosques should continue because prayer can defeat coronavirus disease."[251] It was logical that continuing religious worship should help fight the devil that was COVID-19. It was a position favored by church leaders even where/when they differed with Magufuli's politics,[252] although the pandemic's impact would turn some churches into vaccine centers.

Religious Faiths: Between Organized Religion and Social Distancing

Whereas Christian religious meetings and practices have been widely discussed in the context of COVID-19's spread, and the 'superspreader' nature of religious worship services widely proposed if not articulated, it is useful to consider the complexity of religion in man's life, and to look elsewhere to understand the impact of religious services and festivals such as Hindu and Muslim festivals. Examples of the negative role such religious gatherings have played, increasing the contagion by the pandemic, abound. They include the Sri Petaling religious 'gathering' in Malaysia, which "led to hundreds of COVID-19 cases across Southeast Asia and was directly linked to nearly 35%

Across Multiple Regions in the United States," *JAMA Network Open*, Vol. 4, No. 3 (2021): e212816. doi:10.1001/jamanetworkopen.2021.2816.

[251] Esther Nakkazi, "Obstacles to COVID-19 control in East Africa," *Lancet Infectious Diseases*, Vol. 20, No. 6 (2020): 660. DOI: 10.1016/S1473-3099(20)30382-0.

[252] J. M. Thiga, Impact of COVID-19 Pandemic on the Church's Socioeconomic Well-Being: A Case of Worldwide Gospel Church of Kenya-Githurai Presbytery, I*mpact: Journal of Transformation*, vol. 4, no. 1, (2021), 36-45. Retrieved from https://journals.aiu.ac.ke/index.php/impact/article/view/84.

of cases in Malaysia"[253] Clearly, the virus was no respecter of one, or other religion.

Other outbreaks related to religious festivals occurred in Delhi, India, Iran, and Singapore and even in Saudi Arabia, leading to a closure of mosques all throughout the kingdom while restricting public access to the two holy mosques. Besides guidance by the General Secretariat of the Council of Senior Scholars of Saudi Arabia and the WHO's guidelines on Ramadan, there was concerted effort, elsewhere as well as in Kenya, to limit the potential impact of COVID-19, which may be exacerbated by static religious celebrations, or annual pilgrimages such as the hajj.

By far the most illustrative examples of the impact of pandemics in general and COVID-19 in particular, include religious festivals and other gatherings in India. Although some of those referenced here occurred before COVID-19 obtruded upon the world, festivals such as the Kumbh Mela (in effect translating into the 'serving of the nectar of immortality'), and the attendant "rituals in religious events, such as rolling on the floor, or bathing naked in the river early in the morning, may predispose to skin, respiratory, gastrointestinal and genitourinary infections."[254] Across religions, religious festivals involve a number of rituals, including, for example, a shared sacrament where individuals may drink from the same sources, clearly potentially spreading any viruses that may be present in the faithful.

The challenges of subsuming religion and religious practices to the practical necessities of lockdowns, social distancing and minimizing in-person attendance and contacts among the faithful quickly run into the zealous, sometimes near-fanatical level of faith among adherents. "Although academics and medical professionals might consider mass gatherings such as Kumbh Mela to be blasphemous at this time, many consider this festival to be of non-negotiable religious importance."[255] At the same time, perhaps due to the importance of the religious 'constituency,' public health officials are often loathe to directly challenge the religious impacts of the pandemic.

---

[253] Saber Yezli, and Anas Khan, "COVID-19 pandemic: it is time to temporarily close places of worship and to suspend religious gatherings," *Journal of Travel Medicine*, Vol. 28, No. 2, (March 2021), 1 DOI: 10.1093/jtm/taaa065.

[254] S. Sridhar, P. Gautret and P. Brouqui, "A comprehensive review of the Kumbh Mela: identifying risks for spread of infectious diseases," *Clinical Microbiology and Infection*, Vol. 21, No. 2, (2015), 128, https://doi.org/10.1016/j.cmi.2014.11.021.

[255] Nita Radhakrishnan and Devendra Kumar Gupta, "India's COVID-19 response: science first," The Lancet - Correspondence, Vol. 397, No. 10293 (June 26, 2021), 2464, DOI: https://doi.org/10.1016/S0140-6736(21)01241-1.

The head of Orthopedics at Apollo Hospitals in New Delhi, for instance, acknowledges the seriousness of the second COVID-19 wave, describing it as behaving like a 'Tsunami,' and whose reasons for severity are "easing restrictions by the government and super-spreader events such as election rallies, religious festivals, maha kumbh mela, and weddings [which] have compounded the problem of community spread."[256] However, in the recommendations to defeat the pandemic, Vaishya recommended (1) a speedy implementation of the vaccination campaign and (2) reduction of SARS-CoV-2 transmission through public-health measures' strict enforcement concurrent with the vaccination campaign.[257] Although in-person religious activities are included in the 'public health measures,' spelling them out is useful, considering what the other side is doing. Some religious adherents and spiritual leaders, egged on by the expressed beliefs of such leaders as Tanzania's late president, former US president and Brazilian president Jair Bolsonaro, and some church leaders, the wall of resistance to modifying religious conduct and practices becomes a near-insurmountable COVID-19 stumbling block.

Kenya's, and more broadly, the Global South's COVID-19 fight is also indirectly affected, nay, impeded by religious festivals, congregations and conduct, particularly in India. Prior to the 'delta' surge, "the Serum Institute of India, which is producing the AstraZeneca vaccine (called 'Covishield' in India), was supposed to supply India and export 200 million total doses for distribution via COVAX,"[258] the global compact to help supply vaccines especially to the Global South nations. Delta changed these calculations: "the Indian government has blocked vaccine exports to shore up the domestic supply,"[259] a logical, even expected course of action given the increasing, and previously discussed tendency towards 'vaccine nationalism.' Kenya thus became collateral to India's delta surge.

Absent consistent testing and vaccine supply, prevention becomes one of the most effective ways of dealing with the pandemic. That said, one must keep in mind that Kenya's record of tracking COVID-19 infections, or even testing, is most deplorable. As such, even religious-festival originating COVID-19 clusters are especially difficult, if not impossible to detect, even

---

[256] Raju Vaishya, "The havoc caused by the second wave of COVID-19 in India," *Apollo Medicine* 0;0:0, (28 May, 2021), DOI: 10.4103/am.am_36_21.

[257] Vaishya, "The havoc caused by the second wave," (2021).

[258] Nature Editors, "To curb COVID-19, global health must go local," *Nature medicine*, Vol. 27, No. 929 (2021). https://doi.org/10.1038/s41591-021-01400-y.

[259] Nature Editors, "To curb COVID-19," (2021).

where they occur. It might thus appear that Kenya has been fortunate enough to not have any religious activities that cause COVID surges, but inability to track outcomes is not the same as the outcomes not being present. Still, one would be remiss to suggest that Kenya is somehow special, and that religious festivals do not contribute to contagion or surges. Until better testing is available, this will remain a mystery.

A Non-Negative, Supportive Role of Religion

The role of churches and other religious institutions was not necessarily *only* negative. In fact, for the most part, majority of religions and religious organizations in Kenya, including churches, complied with government directives regarding COVID-19 containment measures. Following suspension of in-person services and meetings, "they maintained worship services, moving them online. They helped Christians make sense of the pandemic and offered themselves as repositories of public trust."[260] Those that had the wherewithal organized various forms of social assistance, such as distribution of food, school supplies and checking in on the faithful and infirm. "Churches are at the forefront of formal and informal health delivery and disease control, through medical services and faith healing."[261]

Even as the government efforts regarding religious services regulation, it was receiving unexpected help from a most unusual source: the National Institutes of Allergies and Infectious Diseases (NIAID) head, Dr. Francis Collins. Appearing on The Late Show with Stephen Colbert, Dr. Francis Collins argued that, "God does a lot of the answer to prayers through people, or through taking careful steps forward."[262] He further gave examples of a Christian putting on a seat belt, or a life-vest on a child who is going swimming, even though the parent prays that God protects the child from drowning. Dr. Collins further noted the compatibility of Christianity and

---

[260] Emma Wild-Wood, Liz Grant, Babatunde Adedibu, Alan Barnard, Aloys Ojore and Yossa Way, "The Public Role of Churches in Early Responses to COVID-19 in Africa: Snapshots from Nigeria, Congo, Kenya and South Africa," *Studies in World Christianity* Vol. 27, No. 1 (2021), 65.

[261] Emma Wild-Wood, et al., "The Public Role of Churches in Early Responses to COVID-19," (2021), 65.

[262] LSSC, "Dr. Francis Collins Discusses The Complexities of Herd Immunity," *The Late Show with Stephen Colbert,* Monday, May 24, 2021, https://web.facebook.com/watch/?extid=SEO----&v=517966956001950; 4:30.

science, noting that for those Christians that ask, "God, where is the answer? Maybe it's through these vaccines."[263]

In his analysis then, there was no fundamental incompatibility between faith and science, and if the science said perhaps keep distance, then that wasn't oppositional to faith since God has also given man the know-how, the ability to invent the internet – perhaps not for the said purposes but also the capacity to stream religious services through the web for the duration of the pandemic. Indeed, one might suspect that doing so might increase the congregation size at no risk.

Without quite articulating their positions in these exact words, religions and organizations carried out their religious and legal obligations, albeit with some grumbling about the differences between crowds in supermarkets, vehicles and political rallies and those in church – a decidedly fair point. Yet in the greater debate, perhaps churches had a point, and neither Dr. Francis Collins nor any author is the authority on matters spiritual, but if following the most important commandment requires social distancing and not attending religious services for a while, then that ought to be the practice.

Socio-Cultural Traditions: Funerals

If (some) African societies are anything to go by, Jean-Baptiste Alphonse Karr's elegant statement, "plus ça change, plus c'est la même chose is absolutely on point. To mangle and perhaps misapply Plato's statement that 'man is a political animal,' the African is a social, communitarian, traditional, socio-cultural and even superstitious being. He has beliefs, traditions, ceremonies, libations, practices, services, prohibitions, celebrations, commiserations, cleansings, and a plethora of sometimes, if not regularly, confounding activities. In scenes that often harkened back to the commitment (or fanaticism) surrounding politics and religion in the context of prohibitions, activities around socio-cultural traditions attracted the same zest, with loud protestations when traditions could not be followed. Think: funerals.

Burials are a necessity, unless one is persuaded by cremation, which most African societies are not, or the more ancient practice of leaving bodies out in the woods, long past. Beyond the possibilities occasioned by potentially not burying the departed, there is a question of dignity. For African societies, it is much more: "several tribes in Kenya believe in life beyond this current life;

[263] LSSC, "Dr. Francis Collins Discusses The Complexities of Herd Immunity," (2021).

[...] this belief in life after death affects the funerals and burial rituals in the community. This is because they are considered to escort the deceased from the world of the living to the spiritual world of the spirits and ancestors."[264] A proper burial is therefore not just necessary; it is self-serving, because otherwise the spirits of the departed might return and 'hover' over the still living. Attendant to the proper burial are rituals and rites, such as "the washing and cleaning of the dead body, the removal of the pant [sic] of the married woman, and set in the position of the reproductive part of the male in case he has left behind a wi[n]dow."[265]

The rest of the world might disagree, even vehemently, with the need to carry out any of these rituals, which decidedly include physical contact with the body and its fluids and given the evidence of the virus surviving for up to 72 hours on surfaces, it was evident that handling such bodies played right into the most efficient method of COVID-19 transmission. Thus, although at the point of Kenya's first COVID-19 case, little was clear about the potential transmission of the virus from bodily fluids of deceased persons, the Kenyan government took immediate and decisive action. But as it is wont to do, in taking decisive actions, they also turned out to be *drastic* – at the beginning of the pandemic, and in subsequent weeks and months. It 'closed public mortuaries and decreed that all bodies were to be buried within 48 hrs, with less than 15 mourners."[266] The disrespect for traditions was inferred during one especially egregious – but by no means the only – case was a burial recorded in the western region of Kenya, for one of the earliest suspected victims of COVID-19:

> The white pickup truck backs out of the darkness into the frame, with several people in white protective suits and facemasks on its open back. They pull a white body bag off the back of the truck, which drops on the ground, is dragged to the grave, and, after short hesitation and intensified wailing by the women in the background, swung into the hole. Going viral on WhatsApp and other social media, it [the video] provoked strong

---

264 Bernard Alwala, "What Has Science to Do with Religion? A Looming Challenge of Traditional and Religious Practices on Curbing the Spread of COVID-19 Pandemic in Kenya," *East African Journal of Traditions, Culture and Religion*, Vol. 2, No. 1, (2020), 22-33 DOI: https://doi.org/10.37284/2707-5370.

265 Alwala, "What has Science to Do with Religion," (2020), 30.

266 P. Wenzel Geissler and Ruth J. Prince, "Layers of epidemy: Present pasts during the first weeks of COVID-19 in western Kenya," *Centaurus*, Vol. 62 No. 2, Spotlight Issue: Histories of epidemics in the time of COVID-19, (May 2020), 248-256, DOI: 10.1111/1600-0498.12295.

emotions across a wide range of people. Even disease control experts, medical professionals, and epidemiologists privately expressed grief and anger. The national outrage forced the Ministry of Health to issue a statement defending the government's actions and propose a protocol for "dignified" burials.[267]

Besides these government-sanctioned burial (or desecration practices), there are less – shock-inducing – practices, but whose impacts are no less significant or deadly. They begin with traditional mourning, occasionally requiring actual wailing in anguish – another outlet for the dreaded aerosolized droplets. Mourning is also a mostly collective affair, conducted in and by groups of people coming in and out of the homestead. By definition, these groups, comprising of many, different sets, are 'superspreader' sites for COVID-19 – after all, besides masks and vaccines, social distancing is the whole game in containing the pandemic's spread.

Mourning is also a multi-day event: in some communities, it occurs over many days, and rotates different people in and out, from relatives to neighbors to well-wishers, some of whom live in different parts of the country. They involve consumption of food, drink and the aforesaid conversations. Absent testing, given the challenge of social distancing and observing other pandemic mitigation strategies, it is exceedingly difficult to assure that contagion will not occur, or know that it has (or has not) occurred. However, we know it does, given similar events in communities outside of Kenya. In addition, because of the limited testing, it is not often clear what the cause of death is, particularly of the decedent. The tendency to 'mishandle' the decedent in the event of unknown causes of death, coupled with the long, asymptomatic incubation period of COVID-19 makes transmission more likely.

COVID-19's danger from funerals does not only arise from improper night-time burials by white-clad government agents; it also includes location. This refers to "home burials, where graves are located within homesteads close to drinking water sources [or] cemeteries and graves located in wetlands and areas with shallow groundwater systems."[268] There is also "rudimentary earth burials of human cadavers wrapped in a blanket or cloth without a coffin […] thereby increasing the risk of groundwater contamination."[269] The first was

---

[267] Geissler and Prince, "Layers of epidemy," (2020), 251.

[268] Willis Gwenzi, "Leaving no stone unturned in light of the COVID-19 faecal-oral hypothesis? A water, sanitation and hygiene (WASH) perspective targeting low-income countries," *Science of The Total Environment*, Vol. 753 (2021), 10, https://doi.org/10.1016/j.scitotenv.2020.141751.

[269] Gwenzi, "Leaving no stone unturned in light of the COVID-19," (2021), 10.

especially evident during India's recent COVID-19 surge between March and June 2021 with burials or body abandonment on the banks of the Ganges and other rivers. In cases where these were not buried by the locals, ultimately, they washed downstream. It is to be remembered that the Ganges, as well as other rivers, are often used for drinking water and for religious purposes, including dipping into the river for cleansing purposes.

A more immediate negative outcome of the contest between the urge to uphold what societal members might consider inviolable traditions with consequences hypothesized to be direr than any possible COVID-19 outcomes particularly given the low death rates, and the government's policy of burial within 72 hours of death, is that community members may actively work against government directives, and in support of local traditions. This includes potentially keeping the sick home (for fear of being diagnosed with COVID-19), hiding victims and failing, or refusing to disclose the cause of death, particularly where COVID-19 is suspected, and thus increasing potential contagion, given the previously discussed limited testing, and almost no-testing of deceased persons.

Indeed, given the ongoing and widespread practice where doctors, afraid that diagnosing "COVID-19" as opposed to "pneumonia" might cause their patients to die from fright (of catching the big one), even COVID-19 deaths are likely to be misreported or underreported – which is already suspected to be widely occurring. If it's not a COVID-19 death, the body may be handled by more people, thus imperiling everyone who mourns, or touches the body. But even the very enforcers of government policy – be they administrators or health officials – often come from the same communities and often hold the same beliefs as the community, over burials and funerals.

The conundrum that faces such government and health ministry personnel is complex. Do they run afoul of government policy by turning a blind eye to customs and traditions? Or do they run afoul of community by strictly enforcing government directives, or both? If they are members of the same communities, they are also likely to be more sympathetic towards the socio-cultural traditions. Thus, ultimately, they may have to enforce directives and decrees they disagree with, or zealously enforce those that they do not agree with, creating hostility towards locals. This is not a useful dilemma to be contending with and may well produce negative outcomes unsupportive of eradicating the pandemic.

Funerary Culture: Constraint or Potential Asset?

It is useful to also take note of positions that contradict the notion that culture can be detrimental to containing the pandemic. For instance, Alwala finds that "by looking at the looming challenges that religion and culture may present to the scientific directives on the spread of COVID-19,"[270] including finding ways to bury the bodies with the proper decorum and dignity, while observing, even designing new community programs that do both: bury properly, and observe the mitigation strategies and restrictions. Paradoxically, though "funerals in Europe and America tend to be private ceremonies while in many communities in Africa they are like public celebrations attended by family, relatives, community and others,"[271] COVID-19 and its high rate of transmissibility is challenging the public nature of funerals, but more importantly, the sheer cost.

Even as friends, relatives and the public mourn, they often end up slaughtering the bereaved family's animals and essentially 'feasting,' a prospect that can easily leave a family destitute, especially if they have repeated burials. Such costs are acknowledged, but justified as demonstrating honor and respect, by celebrating the deceased. Churches especially in western Kenya are ardent advocates against such practices, particularly given that funerals are "the most extravagant of all and the dead is customarily honored on a lavish scale [and] regarded as the largest and outstanding Luo ceremony lasting for days with provisions of food and drinks."[272] Limiting the number of those present at both funerals and mourning, and in the length a body that is kept before being buried (sometimes this is over a week) has clear advantages, at least in the short term. It both reduces the possibility of decreasing the cost of the 'death', and the potential for contagion.

Initiation: Circumcision and FGM

COVID-19's disruptions were not only felt in the most salient of society's actions and activities such as work, education and religious services; it

---

[270] Alwala, "What has Science to Do with Religion," (2020), 33.

[271] Benard Odoyo Okal, Benard Otieno Kodak, Adams Yakub and Jackline Okello, "Implications of Coronavirus (Covid-19) on the Stability of the Luo Cultural Funeral Ceremonies in Kenya," *EAS Journal of Humanities and Cultural Studies*, Vol. 2, No. 2 (Mar-Apr-2020), 96-103, DOI:10.36349/EASJHCS.2020.V02I02.015.

[272] Okal et al. "Implications of Coronavirus," (2020), 100.

affected socio-cultural and life-events as weddings and initiations. Perhaps truly oblivious of the potential impact of their actions, some communities have carried on with other traditions, who's very practice has 'COVID-19 vector' written all over them. One of such long-held and practiced traditions involves initiation, or circumcision, and for women and girls, a more devastating form that is Female Genital Mutilation (FGM).

Circumcision has long been acknowledged as a form of initiation, as one part of the 'rites of passage' in many communities, Kenyan and even external, such as the Jewish people. Whereas initiation is broader in its form (e.g., the removal of six lower teeth among the Luo), circumcision has traditionally been precisely specified, including the when, where, how, and who. Indeed, for most young African, Kenyan men, initiation is the bridge one must cross into adulthood. Besides traditional 'adulthood' functions, medical types of circumcision have increasingly found favor even amongst global health experts, as a way to decrease HIV transmission rates especially in communities with alternative initiation processes.

Some communities have, over time, varied the form and function of circumcision, and this extended in some instances to the centers and medical facilities that carry out the practice. Examples from elsewhere – Zimbabwe in this case – show a closure of even non-traditional, medical facilities serving such purposes, as a result of the onset of the pandemic. "Traditional/religious circumcision camps were shuttered and VMMC (voluntary medical male circumcision) services limited to walk-in only."[273] The closure and re-purposing of medical facilities, churches and schools, which have often served as the sites for alternate rites of passage during school holidays in Kenya deprived most of a safe, better managed, medically-available and potentially less-abusive facilities.

Whether as a rite of passage or alleged religious practice, female circumcision, or female genital mutilation (FGM), on the other hand, is a more contested space, and one whose benefits are suspect at best. It is often described in terms of egregious violation of body autonomy, an expression of paternalism, sexual control and denial, a medically unnecessary practice that is dangerous to the 'victim' – from excessive bleeding to childbirth – and decidedly, as a form of gross human rights violations. It has persisted in Kenya (and overwhelmingly regionally, e.g., in Somalia) is in itself an anathema. It

[273] John Stover, Sherrie L. Kelly, Edinah Mudimu, Dylan Green, Tyler Smith, Isaac Taramusi, Loveleen Bansi-Matharu, Rowan Martin-Hughes, Andrew N. Phillips and Anna Bershteyn, "The Risks and Benefits of Providing HIV Services during the COVID-19 Pandemic," *MedRxiv*, (March 1, 2021), 2 https://doi.org/10.1101/2021.03.01.21252663.

is simultaneously widely practiced by some communities and not others, and claimed as a non-negotiable element of some cultures and peoples.

In recent years, the Kenyan government has articulated a determination to eradicate it, even though doing so risks significant backlash against authorities, as well as accusations of government's lack of respect of cultural traditions, despite the country being a multicultural society comprised of an otherwise diverse populace. During the Nairobi Summit for the International Conference on Population and Development (ICPD 25), co-convened by the Kenyan and Danish governments and UNFPA, Kenya's president Uhuru Kenyatta pledged to eradicate FGM from the country by 2022. And much like the gender agenda of the SDGs under which the Summit was convened, this is a goal that is most unlikely to be accomplished.[274]

Traditions: Rise in FGM Prevalence during COVID-19

The pandemic led to reduced vigilance by government authorities and police in rural areas, even as an influx of Kenyans from cities and urban to rural areas increased and the pandemic worsened amid lockdowns and bans on movement. These deprived many urban dwellers of the means to sustain livelihoods. As the rural numbers swelled, the number of reported FGM cases in some of the rural areas increased, as did the nefariousness and public displays of the practice. For instance, even among the Kikuyu, where the practice is less public and fairly widely frowned upon, several cases made national headlines. They included the violent and forcible initiation of a 38-year-old woman by her husband and 30 of his cohorts. They were allegedly adherents of *mũingĩ-ki* (Mũngĩkĩ), traditional religion practiced among the Kikuyu. The group apparently threatened to visit the same harm upon her daughters.[275] Elsewhere, based on a personal interview with an informant, a reason her husband wanted to divorce her and re-marry was because she would not consent to undergoing FGM.[276]

---

[274] Clara Broekaert, Ceri-Lune Renneboog, Ferdinand Okwaro, Abdu Mohiddin, and Marleen Temmerman, "Working Paper - Digital News Media Coverage on Sexual and Gender-Based Violence in Kenya: Scoping the Impact of the COVID-19 Pandemic," SocArXiv Papers, (2021), 1-15 https://ecommons.aku.edu/eastafrica_fhs_mc_obstet_gynaecol/316.

[275] Alice Waithera, "Men held me down, forcibly cut me - Mũrang'a woman," *The Star – News,* 6th July, 2021, https://www.the-star.co.ke/news/2021-07-05-men-held-me-down-forcibly-cut-me-muranga-woman/.

[276] In-person interview with Peninah Kamau,* 34-year old, mother-of-2, resident of (Tulaga, Kinangop), 08.14. 2021.

Dyer recounts a scene out of the horror shows where "about 2,800 girls from southwestern Kenya's Kuria community who recently underwent female genital mutilation (FGM) have(ing) been paraded through town centers in recent weeks."[277] The trend toward increased cases of FGM has generally held, also among the Maasai. Here, "as a pre-requisite into marriagehood, all the fresh brides have to undergo female genital mutilation (FGM)."[278] COVID-19's onset, the closure of schools, the propensity of some communities to favor educating daughters less, and the decreased level of government surveillance in rural areas repeated among the Maasai, so that FGM instances increased. FGM was already known to most of the girls surveyed (at 95% familiarity), mostly through guardians, NGOs and teachers, with the latter painting the practice negatively.

However, Ole Masago et al., add that "challenges faced by the Maasai girl child which had taken so long to alleviate began re-manifesting themselves back. There was no more school to shelter the girls from teenage pregnancies, FGM [...] economic hardships arising from covid-19 pandemic saw and increase in domestic violence."[279] The particular study also found that "62.1% of the girls had undergone FGM. All the girls initiated indicated that they had been forced to undertake the initiation."[280] Further, "the number of girls undertaking FGM after COVID-19 had sharply risen [based on] more free time at home and less intrusion of the culture by formal education and NGOs,"[281] giving parents and guardians more leeway; clearly, COVID-19 has been more harmful to girls. This holds, even though the practice – from cutting to celebration thereof – serves as veritable disease vectors.

Two developments make the honor roll: perceived overall decrease of FGM incidents even with the decrease in monitoring and therewith, ability to get away executing the practice, and the increasing medicalization of FGM. The former conceals the numbers on pervasiveness: "about 4 million females

---

277 Owen Dyer, "FGM: nearly 3000 girls are paraded in Kenya as pandemic hinders control efforts," *BMJ: British Medical Journal (Online)*; Vol. 371, (Oct 28, 2020), n.p. doi:10.1136/bmj.m416.

278 Morompi Ole Masago, Bakari Chaka, Kelele Joshua Sambu Alice, Jebet Sheila, and G. Reuben, "Effects of Covid-19 Pandemic on the Welfare of the Maasai Girl Child in Narok County, Kenya," *European Journal of Social Sciences*, Vol. 3, No. 3, (2020), 124 http://hdl.handle.net/123456789/11071.

279 Ole Masago, et al., "Effects of Covid-19 Pandemic on the Welfare of the Maasai Girl Child," (2020), 125.

280 Ole Masago, et al., "Effects of Covid-19 Pandemic on the Welfare of the Maasai Girl Child," (2020), 137.

281 Ole Masago, et al., "Effects of Covid-19 Pandemic on the Welfare of the Maasai Girl Child," (2020), 137.

in Kenya have undergone the cut, translating to 21% of the victims, with ages ranging from 15 to 49 years."[282] In actual numbers, this computes to 4 million women and girls. Those most likely to undergo the practice are in the north-eastern region of the country at 98%, the practice with described as near universal, while those least likely to be subject to the practice are more likely to live in the Rift Valley, Central, Western and Coast provinces of Kenya.[283] UNICEF projections on the 'percentage of adolescent girls aged 15 to 19 years who are expected to undergo FGM' at the pace of current progress, suggests that the practice will peter out to 0% girls by 2050.[284]

On the second issue, FGM has undergone some modifications including medicalizing the process. This may alleviate some of the suffering and the deaths that inevitably occur during, and post-FGM process. However, they in no way take away from its needlessness, the invasion of privacy, the loss of autonomy, human rights violations and the other outcomes that have been associated with FGM. According to UNICEF, "seven out of ten girls are circumcised by traditional practitioners, who often use crude tools, while the rest undergo medicalised FGM."[285] However, according to the UNFPA, among the countries in which FGM is performed by medical professionals, Kenya ranks third from the bottom, in Africa, with 15% of such cases.[286]

This would then suggest that 85% of the mutilations are performed by untrained individuals who are likely to use unsanitized instruments, not only elevating the risk of HIV and other diseases being transmitted, but also COVID-19. More presciently, one shudders to think of what the pandemic has done to these numbers. Considering that the national, and devolved governments shuttered some facilities and re-designated others as COVID-19 units, and the dearth of PPE to facilitate safe medical procedures – even of the FGM kind – non-professional medical procedures continue to increase peril to FGM victims. Procedures carried out by traditionalists are more likely to attract local celebrations, another potential pathway for COVID-19 transmission. It can be concluded then, that in the summary, COVID-19 has increased the performance of FGM, the potential for its transmission, and

---

[282] UNICEF, "A Profile of Female Genital Mutilation in Kenya," *UNICEF*, 2020. http://data.unicef.org/wp-content/Fuploads/Profile-of-FGM-in-Kenya-English_2020.pdf.

[283] UNICEF, "A Profile of Female Genital Mutilation in Kenya," (2020), 21.

[284] UNICEF, "A Profile of Female Genital Mutilation in Kenya," (2020), 23.

[285] UNICEF, "A Profile of Female Genital Mutilation in Kenya," (2020), 6.

[286] UNFPA, "Female genital mutilation (FGM) frequently asked questions," United Nations Population Fund, July 2020, https://www.unfpa.org/resources/female-genital-mutilation-fgm-frequently-asked-questions.

complicated local societal and governmental attempts to eradicate the pandemic.

Weddings, Bride-Price/Wealth and Other Celebratory Occasions

Celebrations of new union, such as weddings and the less formal traditional marriage ceremonies are, have also been traditionally large group affairs, in what one might describe as a preening activity – after all, marriage takes place long before the very public ceremony to which individuals are invited to feast and celebrate and mingle, another COVID-19 vector. Weddings especially abroad – and again, here, it is for the lack of widespread testing in Kenya and so, data is lacking on the impact of such events – weddings have been some of the major sources of so-called 'clusters.' However, as alluded to earlier, considering evidence from a number of Kenya's seroprevalence studies, it is clear that COVID-19 has spread widely even absent testing.

Dowry and bride-price payment among the more tradition-adhering is a most interesting phenomenon, particularly with regard to the ceremonies. There are frequent interactions in practically every instance. The ceremonies and other festivals are described by African scholars (countering Finnegan's (1970) argument), as being "fully dramatic and literary."[287] However the ceremonies differ, they are integrative and sequential. For example, among the Kipsigis (some include the Tugen) who practice Koito (a formal drama related to marriage and one that 'defines the Tugen people, sustained by future generations,' the process "begins while the girls are in the initiation; that is when the father of the forthcoming groom pays a formal visit to the father of the young lady he wants for his child."[288]

Notwithstanding the COVID-19 pandemic, one almost understands the continued need to carry out the festival. "Acceptable behaviors in the society are communicated through Koito traditional performances like songs and oral narratives."[289] The necessity of continuing the basic elements of society, through ceremonies and such, stands in contrast to the destructive nature and

[287] Janet J. Kangogo, "The Elements of Drama in *Koito* a Traditional Wedding Ceremony Among the Tugen People of Baringo Kenya," *CHSS Thesis and Dissertations – UoN Digital Repository*, UoN Research Archive, (2020), http://erepository.uonbi.ac.ke/handle/11295/154605.

[288] Kangogo, "The Elements of Drama in Koito," (2020), 31.

[289] Kangogo, "The Elements of Drama in Koito," (2020), 3.

power of the pandemic, and not reconciled. Some other examples of the performative nature of bride-price are captured all throughout the region. Among the Nandi, the "parents of the young man go to the home of the girl's parents."[290] They are usually accompanied by a retinue of family, friends and relatives of married age and good repute as they make entreaties on behalf of their son. Later, an "elaborate ceremonial [...] takes place,"[291] and just as regularly a marriage is "sealed by a final ceremony."[292] Among the 'Waniaturu', "the marriage is finally consummated with ceremonies occurring upon the delivery of these cattle."[293]

Today, bride-price and bride-wealth may take less of the format of cows, sheep and goats and more of money, but it is nonetheless an important element of society and how individuals and societies conceive of themselves. Additionally, though the intensity of these types of ceremonies has decreased somewhat over time, betrothal, marriage, dowry and bride-wealth exchanges, naming and celebration of new births, and their attendant, elaborate ceremonies, continue to occur. Because most of the ceremonies are just as often small-group activities and rarely meet the 50-person threshold that the government generally forbids from meeting during the pandemic, they continue unabated and unsupervised. One cannot under-estimate the impact of the small, intimate gatherings – in Kenya and elsewhere – as incubator spaces for the COVID-19 pandemic.

Harambees: Pulling Together or Pooling Contagion?

The other most Kenyan practice that has been significantly impacted in confound ways is 'Harambee.' Harambee is a concept thought to date back to 1899, during the construction of the Kenya-Uganda railway. Then, the so-called Indian 'coolies' (railway builders) would appeal to one of the Hindu gods for strength – or so the story goes. In post-independence Kenya, it came to take on the essence of the nation and became as Kenyan as the 3,000-metre steeplechase. It was especially given meaning and importance by the Kenya's first president, Jomo Kenyatta, and it featured prominently even on Kenya's coat of arms. It was designed to be part of the national consciousness, a project

[290] Melville J. Herskovits, "The Cattle Complex in East Africa," *American Anthropologist*, New Series, Vol. 28, No. 1 (Jan. - Mar., 1926): 364 https://www.jstor.org/stable/660813.
[291] Herskovits, "The Cattle Complex in East Africa," (1926), 364.
[292] Herskovits, "The Cattle Complex in East Africa," (1926), 365.
[293] Herskovits, "The Cattle Complex in East Africa," (1926), 364.

that appears to have succeeded wildly. Defined as "a Kiswahili word meaning 'pulling together,' [it] invokes the spirit of self-help amongst Kenyans."[294]

Historically, Harambee has been credited with many accomplishments in areas of education (building schools and purchasing educational materials), health (building dispensaries and health centers) and on the environmental front (building gabions to stem runoffs, planting trees, etc.,) among other collective endeavors. But over the years, its use has expanded to include private and individual uses such as paying hospital fees, raising school fees, collective labor to assist in building especially adobe houses, burials and even raising money for dowry and to pay for Christian weddings. Harambee has also featured prominently in the Kenyan political scene, with leaders using the Harambee as an opportunity to meet the public and constituents, to plan their runs for office, and occasionally, to flaunt their wealth.

Even during the pandemic, the practice has not died or diminished. While the bulk of Harambees have continued in the traditional, in-person activities notwithstanding the limits on in-person meetings, there is also an online component that leverages social media platforms such as MChanga and the more global version of GoFundMe, among others.[295] Simultaneously, even though it is essentially African communitarian practice to live in community, there are those who go door-to-door to provide food and other assistance, including assistance coming into the country from the Diaspora.

These activities that draw upon these "local traditions, such as the tradition of 'harambee' community self-help events in Kenya […] have made effective use of social media"[296] while retaining elements of the traditional in-person meetings. Belying the pandemic realities, the in-person meetings continue to increase the risk to Kenyans especially as the Delta variant continues to upend a world that assumed the battle against COVID-19 was almost won. On the same Harambee front, Kenyan businesses have also been active, visible and instrumental in providing support very publicly, donating to support different causes and groups, giving away food, supplies and on

---

[294] A. V. Noreh, "Harambee in Kenya: A Bibliography," October, 1968, University of Nairobi Library, http://erepository.uonbi.ac.ke/bitstream/handle/11295/40009/Norey%20A.%20V.pdf?sequence=1.

[295] Nkirote Laiboni, "Kenya's Philanthropic Tradition Tackles the COVID-19 Challenge," *Coronavirus Response: Chatham House* (9 June 2020), https://www.chathamhouse.org/2020/06/kenyas-philanthropic-tradition-tackles-covid-19-challenge.

[296] Ralph Hamann, Judy N. Muthuri, Ijeoma Nwagwu, Neeveditah Pariag-Maraye, Wendy Chamberlin, Shivani Ghai and Kenneth Amaeshi, "COVID-19 in Africa: Contextualizing Impacts, Responses, and Prospects," *Environment: Science and Policy for Sustainable Development*, Vol. 62, No. 6, (2020): 8-18 – Where Do We Go From Here? Reframing Sustainability for a Post-COVID-19 Era https://doi.org/10.1080/00139157.2020.1820293.

occasion, PPE and other in-demand medical supplies, thus supplementing some of the work done by philanthropic groups, NGOs and even individuals.[297]

One additional pandemic impact on the tradition of giving is worth mentioning. Harambee, depends on having a surplus to give to others. The pandemic's impact on disposable income, and the pressure it has put on households, has led to adaptations. To meet all expenditures with reduced income, households "gave out less gifts and remittances themselves, lent less money to others and postponed loan repayments […] significantly reduced expenditures on schooling and transportation" and otherwise kept expenditures low, but "at the cost of reduced informal risk-sharing and social support between households."[298] The duality of the impact of the pandemic is thus clear: while giving and contributing to aid one's fellow man continues, some modifications have become necessary.

Some Thoroughly Confusing Considerations

Highly centralized and communitarian societies are a key feature of the modern African nation. Kenya boasts of 43 different ethnic groups, each with their traditions, beliefs, ceremonies and their attendant peculiarities. Many of these are highly social events, with interpersonal interactions between and among the members of the community. Even in a modernized country, the level of fidelity to the traditions is quite high, and society members propose all manner of negative outcomes if the social and cultural traditions are not followed as specified. These include, for example, allegedly being haunted by spirits if the dead are not properly buried, including with feasting, eating, drinking and dance. Social and cultural traditional activities are taken seriously.

Additional reasons thereto are self-evident. Because identity is all that more important, public signaling of those activities that confer, affirm or remove identity are equally important, and unlikely to be derailed by a pandemic. In fact, reports of secret circumcision and FGM ceremonies were

---

[297] Hamann, et al., "COVID-19 in Africa," (2020): 14.

[298] Wendy Janssens, Menno Pradhan, Richard de Groot, Estelle Sidze, Hermann Donfouet, and Amanuel Abajobir. "The short-term economic effects of COVID-19 and risk-coping strategies of low-income households in Kenya: A rapid analysis using weekly financial household data." *Tinbergen Institute Discussion Paper*, TI 2020-040/V, Tinbergen Institute, 2020, http://dx.doi.org/10.2139/ssrn.3640340.

that violated the bans against gathering, were rife. Troublingly, not many communities or ceremonies foresaw the potential need for alternatives if and when people could not meet in person. As such, the choices were either to carry out the festivals and ceremonies, or not at al. Most communities could not countenance carrying out the ceremonies, further imperiling the public health of the communities. That contrarian actions by government officers and politicians were not helping is beyond doubt.

Alongside the socio-cultural and traditional community activities, religion, religious belief and the faithful observance of religious faith, services, activities and ceremonies is equally, if not more important. Especially in a time of seemingly intractable misery and death, often alone due to the social distancing requirements, faith became a most important go-to source of solace and support. The inability to meet in person, while well-intentioned, also suffered from the same lack of technology that other endeavors did. Further, most of those who identify as more religious are likely to be older, and less able to work with technology (which in the case of Kenya, was less so available), thus further compounding the negatives. Kenya's lockdown rules almost necessarily discriminated against especially the elderly: the government strongly recommended (if not banned) the attendance of social events and religious services by those over the age of 55 (58). Not only did this rob them of great spiritual support and community, but it also threatened to further increase the isolation that especially the vulnerable persons and groups were already experiencing.

The road to hell is often said to be paved with the best intentions. However, we must recognize that as flawed as the social distancing, lockdown and limits on in-person gatherings were, the scant knowledge that exited in the initial period of the virus' spread often led to leaders wielding a hammer and seeing every small issue as a nail. The limitations on in=person gatherings were rarely ever enforced, and especially supermarkets in Kenya were more notorious for packing in clients, without adhering to the capacity limits. In the context of jobs being lost and no government income replacement schemes, one can almost see the reason for the thinking. At the same time, it led to allegations of discrimination against religious beliefs, and even suggestions that he leaders would burn in hell for their choices. One was almost inclined to agree, considering that the leaders themselves acted as if COVID-19 did not exist, particularly when they were out and about popularizing the BBI Imitative.

Chapter 7

COVID-19 Mitigation Strategies, Implications and Outcomes

Abstract

This chapter broadly examines the various mitigation strategies that the Kenyan government has recommended, adopted and implemented, focusing on the gendered aspects of the pandemic. The nature of Kenyan society and the role of women as caregivers in all instances, has often exposed women to more marginal outcomes while caring for the sick, but also, the effects of the lockdowns on women who are often the primary providers. It examines the implications for the chosen strategies and the outcomes achieved. It comprehensively deals with several specific issues: the impact of the pandemic on gender and exacerbating inequality, the impact on overall food security particularly on women and vulnerable populations needing to both shelter in place and assure access to food, overall nutrition and wellness, the pandemic's impact on human development and poverty, health, health, healthcare and access, the impact on personal security, human security, on governance and on government. The chapter proposes some strategies for increased effectiveness of the mitigation, without further exacerbating the vulnerability of marginalized populations.

Exacerbating Gender (In)-Equality in the Age of COVID-19

It would be remiss not to consider COVID-19's impact and implications on gender in Kenya. More specifically, it is necessary to consider the relationship between COVID-19's onset and persistence and implications for gender and (in)equality. For as much as there has been significant focus on the boy-child on account of increasing evidence that the boy child is increasingly neglected as the world's focus shifts squarely towards the girl child, women are still treated as second-class citizens. In Kenya and more broadly, around Africa, women are far worse off, pummeled by both ethnic and linguistic group marginalization, and also by state policy that is capable of disenfranchising them or fail to correct the disenfranchisement, with two major issues being inheritance and often, not educating the girl child.

There is general consensus that in most societies around the world, women are treated different than men, across a range of variables: equal opportunity, property ownership, leadership opportunities, ability to choose their own future and a myriad of other fronts. Kenya is no different; it struggles between the national and the communal, a most delicate dance. What to do about gender equality is another especially contested space, even with countries that are signatories to global conventions that promise, and hopefully attempt, to achieve equality. For even within the obvious inequality (oppression, even) of women, some assert that this is the proper place of women. But, inequality has implications for humanity, now exacerbated by COVID-19.

It is especially useful to consider Kenyan women and girls' experiences in the context of the Gender Inequality Index (GII). Although data from 2020 and 2021 is not available, and the last available data year and report are from 2019, it is evident from the foregoing that these two groups were especially (negatively) impacted by the pandemic. The GII is associated with such concepts and measures as 'access to opportunities,' and not the actual levels of resources and opportunities in countries; 'outcomes, rather than inputs of means', and 'proximity to gender equality rather than women's empowerment."[299] More specifically, GII measures "the gap between men and women across four fundamental categories (subindexes): Economic Participation and Opportunity, Educational Attainment, Health and Survival and Political Empowerment."[300]

Across the world, the gender gap stands at about 0.68 from the most recent data, and has stagnated there for a several years. Kenya's 2018 GII score was 0.671 (scores range from 0 to 1, with 1 being the most equal, or least difference). Kenya was ranked 109th globally, its score below the slightly improved, global average 'distance' in gender inequality data point of 68.6%[301] – although the Equal Measures 2030 compact and data-set computes this score at 65.7.[302] The 2018 score reflected a -33, negative rank change, indicating

---

[299] World Economic Forum, *Measuring the Global Gender Gap*, (Geneva: The World Economic Forum, 2021). https://reports.weforum.org/global-gender-gap-report-2018/measuring-the-global-gender-gap/?doing_wp_cron=1629014648.401953935623168 9453125.

[300] World Economic Forum, *Global Gender Gap Report 2020,* (Geneva: The World Economic Forum, 2019), 5. URL: http://www3.weforum.org/docs/WEF_GGGR_2020.pdf.

[301] World Economic Forum, *Global Gender Gap Report 2020*, (2019), 9.

[302] Equal Measures 2030, "Harnessing The Power of Data for Gender Equality – Introducing the 2019 EM2030 SDG Gender Index," Equal Measures 2030, (2019), 15 Data:

that over time, Kenya was doing worse in terms of gender equality. The GII score is also indicated to have declined by 0.029 points.

The United Nations – specifically, UNDP data – paints an even direr picture. In its (then) most recent statistical update of the 2019 Gender Inequality Index, Kenya ranked 134th with a GII value of 0.545 based on SDGs 3.1 (maternal mortality ratio), SDG 3.7 (adolescent birth rate), SDG 5.5 (share of seats in parliament), SDG 4.6 (population with some HS education) and labor participation rates.[303] Given that WEF estimates that the global gender 'distance' gap will close in 99 years, one anticipates then, that Kenya's gender inequality gap will close much later: it will take more than a century for Kenyan women and girls to achieve gender equality.[304] And there is little reason to think that when post-COVID-19 GII is computed, Kenya will show any improvements in ranking or score, given the clear negative impacts that the pandemic has had on the two groups, as discussed elsewhere in this volume.

Findings from the SDG Gender Index, conceived by Equal Measures 2030 (EM2030), ostensibly to develop "tools to support data-driven analysis and to hold governments accountable for gender equality in the context of"[305] SDGs, show a middling level of achievement in Kenya's progress towards gender equality. In the report, Kenya performed better than 75% of the other countries in one category: the percentage and rates of women who use digital banking.[306] However, in the '2019 SDG Gender Index scores and rankings by country,' it is ranked 97th of 129 countries in the overall Gender Index, placing it in the bottom 25%. Its score of 55.1 is marginal at best, pitted against better performers and higher ranked nations, e.g., Norway's 89.3.[307] Then again, some countries do assure the equal treatment of all their citizens.

Another (of the few) bright spots is that Kenya is ranked 8th in Sub-Saharan Africa, out of the 33 countries in the region for which data is available.[308] Most of its SDG GII scores are below 60, except for SDG#2 (hunger and nutrition) and SDG#8 (work and economic growth), where it has

---

www.data.em2030.org/2019-global-report; URL: https://www.equalmeasures2030.org/wp-content/uploads/2019/07/EM2030_2019_Global_Report_English_WEB.pdf.

303 UNDP, "Gender Inequality Index," Human Development Indices: A statistical update 2019 | *United Nations Development Programme | UN Data*, Last updated June 2nd, 2020, http://data.un.org/DocumentData.aspx?id=415.

304 World Economic Forum, *Global Gender Gap Report 2020*, (2019), 9.

305 Equal Measures 2030, "SDG Gender Index," *Equal Measures 2030 | Gender Advocates Data Hub, 2021*, https://www.equalmeasures2030.org/products/sdg-gender-index/.

306 Equal Measures 2030, "Harnessing the Power of data for Gender Equality," (2019), 9.

307 Equal Measures 2030, "Harnessing the power of data," (2019), 13.

308 Equal Measures 2030, "Harnessing the Power of data," (2019), 40.

made some progress towards equality.[309] Notwithstanding, Kenya's overall near stagnation is not a proud accomplishment even though it is doing better than other African countries. This is pertinent given that "with an average regional index score of 51.1, the Sub-Saharan Africa region is the lowest scoring region overall in the 2019 SDG Gender Index."[310] Kenya is doing okay but only amongst a low-scoring group. It is an unenviable position, akin to being a mid-size fish in a very small pond.

In terms of the impact of pandemic mitigation measures, women came off worse than men. For instance, women reported skipping meals 6% more than men, 15% more likely to have lost income, 8% more likely to experience domestic and intimate partner violence (household violence) and 6% more likely to under-utilize, or fail to utilize healthcare at all than men.[311] Other preliminary reports and projections align with these expectations. Based on previous data and evidence following other health crises, "there is evidence to suggest that women and girls in SSA will suffer from extreme and multifaceted negative secondary impact as a result of the COVID-19 crisis"[312] in such areas as girls' education, social protection, unintended pregnancies, healthcare access, poverty, livelihood, land rights, women and girls' employment (formal or other), food security and nutrition, political leadership, child marriage, rights, empowerment and even political participation.[313] It is evident, then, that COVID-19 stands to negatively, massively impact women.

Besides the tangible economic disadvantages that have been visited upon women and girls' lives to even include personal well-being, there have been more intimate, intensely personal downsides to rights to personhood and the security of the person. These effects do not merely refer to the sometimes abstract, data-driven concepts of an ~X~ percentage 'decrease in overall welfare.' Rather, the outcomes include an increase in domestic, homebound,

---

[309] Equal Masures 2030, "2019 SDG Gender Index: Key Findings," *Equal Measures 2030 Data Hub*, August 2021, https://data.em2030.org/2019-sdg-gender-index/key-findings/.

[310] Equal Measures 2030, "Harnessing the Power of data," (2019), 41.

[311] Karen Austrian, Nandita Rajshekhar, Timothy Abuya, Beth Kangwana, Rhoune Ochako, Benjamin Tidwell, Daniel Mwanga, Eva Muluve, Faith Mbushi, Mercy Nzioki, and Thoai D Ngo, "Gendered economic, social and health effects of the COVID-19 pandemic and mitigation policies in Kenya: evidence from a prospective cohort survey in Nairobi informal settlements," *British Medical Journal (BMJ) Open* (2021);11:e042749. doi: 10.1136/bmjopen-2020-042749.

[312] Rafaeli, Tal and Geraldine Hutchinson, "The Secondary Impacts of COVID-19 on Women and Girls in Sub-Saharan Africa," *K4D Helpdesk Report 830*, (2020). Brighton, UK: Institute of Development Studies. https://opendocs.ids.ac.uk/opendocs/handle/20.500.12413/15408.

[313] Rafaeli and Hutchinson, "The Secondary Impacts of COVID-19," (2020).

intimate partner (IPV) and gender-based violence (GBV). Kenya government's *ad hoc* responses to the increase in gendered violence, coupled with the more general "lack[ing] [of] sector-specific guidelines to ensure availability of comprehensive GBV services and programmes"[314] further assure that women's lot is going to be worse off, perhaps reversing any gains achieved before COVID-19 began. Calls to address mental health crises that are increasingly more violent and are largely tied to deadly domestic violence have elicited little in way of policy responses. One hopes that some policy wonk somewhere is crafting a response, a national strategy.

There exists other less obvious COVID-19 impacts on women, especially in the delivery of healthcare. Although the Kenyan government waived all maternity fees, the parallel designation of COVID-19 hospitals reduced capacity as to where women can access these free pre- and post-natal services. Home births have increased (and persisted in some hard-to-reach communities), where midwives help with delivery of children. COVID-19 compounded some reproductive health challenges by leading an increase in teenage pregnancies and overall "unintended pregnancies resulting from reduced attendance for contraception due to fear of exposure to COVID-19 at health facilities."[315]

Midwives who help to deliver babies face increased risks of maternal and infant mortality, and unsafe deliveries, which may increase the probability of catching COVID-19 and transmitting onward to their own families much as has been the case with first responders e.g., the police. Besides the trend that has seen many women increasingly shunning reproductive health facilities due to the aforementioned risks, there is loss of community-based healthcare, which has often been considered more effective than state managed healthcare and reproductive health services.

This is because "midwives play a key role in contraception counselling and addressing the socio-cultural myths related to extremely low levels of use of family planning,"[316] services, and non-consultation declines these possibilities. These findings were especially evident in Kenya, Uganda and Tanzania. Research finds that "cases of infection have been reported amongst

---

[314] Neetu John, Charlotte Roy, Mary Mwangi, Neha Raval and Terry McGovern, "COVID-19 and gender-based violence (GBV): hard-to-reach women and girls, services, and programmes in Kenya," *Gender & Development*, Vol. 29, No. 1 (2021), 55-71, DOI: 10.1080/13552074.2021.1885219.

[315] Eunice Pallangyo, Mary Grace Nakate, Rose Maina, and Valerie Fleming, "The impact of covid-19 on midwives' practice in Kenya, Uganda and Tanzania: A reflective account," *Midwifery*, 89, (Oct. 2020), 102775. doi: 10.1016/j.midw.2020.102775.

[316] Pallangyo, et al., "The impact of covid-19 on midwives' practice," (2020).

midwives and other healthcare personnel."[317] Thus, even as women continue with the important, albeit dangerous work, and as pandemic job loss almost doubles that of men, computing to an estimated 43%[318] of all COVID-19 job losses, *and* continues to be paid less, the work they do is ever more important.

A brief discussion on the impact of COVID-19 on health, healthcare access and the pandemic's impact on NTDs and other common illnesses in Kenya is in the next section. However, it is useful to briefly highlight evidence and findings from several African countries including Kenya, of the specific ways in which COVID-19 has affected women and revealed itself to be highly gendered. Such findings show a "decline in the ability to see a health-care provider since March 2020 [being] greater for women than for men" and the role that higher levels of education played (more educated women were more likely to seek medical care despite the pandemic).[319] It is clear that COVID-19 is a highly gendered pandemic, one which, in the final analysis, will have diminished any of the gains that gender equity programs and efforts have made so far, absent concerted, strategic government planning, programs and interventions, currently and in the waning days of the pandemic.

Effects on Food Security, Nutrition and Wellness

Some of the other COVID-19 impacts are deeply personal, even though they are shared by millions across the country. Nutrition and wellness are especially important because as seen previously, lack of adequate nutrition leads to undernutrition, malnutrition, delayed development, occasional stunting, and life-long health complications and ultimately, lower life expectancy and lower overall but especially economic productivity. These negative preparatory factors portend, and procure further negative outcomes for the long-term human resource and individual development possibilities. Indeed, one can argue that inadequate nutrition leads to not only underdevelopment, but long-

---

[317] Pallangyo, et al., "The impact of covid-19 on midwives' practice," (2020).

[318] Anu Madgavkar, Olivia White, Mekala Krishnan, Deepa Mahajan, and Xavier Azcue, "COVID-19 and gender equality: Countering the regressive effects," *McKinsey Global Institute*, (July 2020), 2, https://www.apucis.com/frontend-assets/porto/initial-reports/COVID-19-and-gender-equality-Countering-the-regressive-effects-vF.pdf.pagespeed.ce.DDg-UdcoaA.pdf.

[319] Safa Abdalla, Elizabeth G Katz, and Gary L Darmstadt, "Gender and the impact of COVID-19 on demand for and access to health care: analysis of data from Kenya, Nigeria, and South Africa," *The Lancet - Global Health* – Special Issue, Vol. 9, No., S7, (March 01, 2021) DOI: https://doi.org/10.1016/S2214-109X(21)00115-7.

term loss of human resource capacity due to frail, sickly and weak citizens. But the insufficient and poor nutrition practices have more immediate and (im)-practical implications: it is unfathomable that even a well-meaning government can enforce movement bans, lockdowns and curfews at the risk of citizens' starvation. Governments rarely do well in food fights with citizens, as Louis XIV found out, and as many subsequent governments have since.

The basis of foundation of government is to secure the welfare of citizens. Because citizens are not at liberty to live under *no government*, the relationship between them and the government is thus a contract. It is not the government's job to provide food or other basic necessities; however, the citizens' contract with government requires it to make possible the conditions to search for livelihoods – and welfare. This includes *not* limiting their ability to provide for their livelihoods, without giving alternatives. Government's provision of food during crisis conditions is not only in the interest of its own survival and the health of the citizens; it is also in the interest of ensuring that curfews and quarantines will not be violated *because* citizens are looking for food. After all, given the numbers (deaths from malnutrition and hunger versus from COVID-19), the latter wins hands-down.

Most studies done during the past 15 months or so have shown negative food and nutritional outcomes preceding, but also being the result of the COVID-19 pandemic. For instance, food *insecurity* in Kenya and Uganda increased by 38% and 44% respectively, while fruit consumption reportedly decreased by 30% since the advent of COVID-19. Across most developing countries and specifically Kenya, a 4.2% food price increase was recorded in in March alone.[320] Reflecting other findings on the state of poverty and hunger in the world, COVID-19's impact on two vulnerable groups, women and children, is also more severe and negative. Generally, it is estimated that women and girls account for 60% of all under-nourished persons in the world, while 70% of the 1.3 billion people who live in poverty worldwide are women.[321] But that is not the only challenge. WFP (USA), with concurrence by World Hunger, notes that in some cultures, "women [are still expected to] often eat last and least in countries facing conflict, famine and hunger" even

[320] Endashaw Workie, Joby Mackolil, Joan Nyika and Sendhil Ramadas, "Deciphering the impact of COVID-19 pandemic on food security, agriculture, and livelihoods: A review of the evidence from developing countries," *Current Research in Environmental Sustainability*, Vol. 2, (2020), https://doi.org/10.1016/j.crsust.2020.100014.

[321] World Hunger, "Women and Hunger Facts," World Hunger Education Service, (2020), https://www.worldhunger.org/women-and-hunger-facts/.

though they are also likely to do the most amount of work.[322] Specific to Kenya's case, approximately 12 million women and girls classified as undernourished.[323]

There was an additional phenomenon that arose out of the pandemic's earliest ravages and the steps the Kenyan government took to address it: urban-rural flight. This led to the creation of multi-generational households, but also put pressure on the food supplies. For example, the author's two sisters, with their (total eight) children, relocated from Nairobi to the area around Naivasha; many other Kenyans departed urban areas to rural areas. This almost reversed the usual practice where those in urban areas are more likely to contribute to the welfare of those in the rural areas. The closure of many businesses and therewith, sources of income, meant that not only was the usual support missing; urbanites relocating to the rural areas implied a double negative. Urban-rural relocations put more pressure on the food supply, and without any significant change in food production capacity, or government assistance, the negative effects continued to manifest.

Kenyan government's response (or lack thereof) smacks of an absence of any coherent strategies to deal with food security, (mal) nutrition and hunger. Slammed by the quadruple whammy – the 2019 and subsequently recurrent locust infestations, perennial drought, lack of food especially in the ASAL areas, the impact of COVID-19 and the trickle-down maleficent effects of poverty, the government ought to have implemented a strategy that might ensure food security, beyond the measly Kshs. 13 per month that it provided for citizens at high risk of food insecurity at the beginning of the pandemic. Add that measly amount to the corruption that sees even food assistance diverted and used as political incentives and, or cudgels, the incoherence of the (non-existent) strategy is staggering.

Human Development Implications and Impact on Poverty

Although it may be too early to determine the full-spectrum impact of COVID-19 on human development and its measures, it is clear that the major HDI indicators, i.e., life expectancy, education and per capita income have been

[322] World Food Program USA, "Women are hungrier," *World Food Program USA, 2021*, https://www.wfpusa.org/women-are-hungrier-infographic/.

[323] Max Roser and Hannah Ritchie, "Hunger and Undernourishment," (2019) *Published online at OurWorldInData.org.* Retrieved from: 'https://ourworldindata.org/hunger-and-undernourishment' [Online Resource].

negatively impacted. One expects to find that the levels of poverty have increased as the per capita income decreases due to the lockdowns and closure of businesses, while the time that most learners have spent outside of school has had a deleterious impact on achievement, human security, food nutrition, safety from abuse and exploitation, and a plethora of other negative outcomes that are often associated with learners being out of school, but especially considering the Kenyan context where most secondary school students often attend boarding schools.

Without a doubt, COVID-19 has led to an increase in poverty levels with significant effects being especially felt by women, children and youth. These are groups that the Kenyan government has recently identified as being either minority or vulnerable – when more than 70% of a country is populated by the minority and vulnerable groups, it is quite the challenge. Increased poverty levels correlate negatively with well-being, and with life expectancy. Poverty and poor nutrition lead to further negative outcomes with regard to food and nutrition, which may be exacerbated by existing vulnerabilities to disease. One surmises that all these issues are interconnected: insufficient food leads to poor health outcomes, poor health outcomes diminish the quality of life and can contribute to chronic illnesses, while illnesses have the capacity to reduce life expectancy. All these variables are present in Kenya during the pandemic.

Mitigation strategies, if properly, fairly and competently implemented, had the chance to see to it that the burden was decreased. For countries such as Kenya, which do not have formal, social security and social protection infrastructure (the 'pesa ya wazee' concept is ill implemented and there is not a systematic approach to disseminating the money to all eligible citizens, despite most having mobile phones and M-PESA), COVID-19 has also exposed the vulnerability of the elderly population. Most poverty is anticipated to reside among women and girls (and more generally, youth), but increasingly, evidence shows that older Kenyans, who are unlikely to be able to provide for themselves through (especially agricultural) labor, are in the cross-hairs of growing levels of poverty.

One gem of a potentially bright spot was the study finding that "chronic disease was not appreciably more-affected by inequality [...] suggesting that inequality as such may not be an important determinant of health even for chronic disease."[324] Simultaneously, another research study, while indirectly

[324] Brian Biggs, Lawrence King, Sanjay Basu and, David Stuckler, "Is wealthier always healthier? The impact of national income level, inequality, and poverty on public health in Latin America," *Social Science & Medicine*, Vol. 71, No. 2, (2010): 266-273, https://doi.org/10.1016/j.socscimed.2010.04.002.

addressing inequality, found “a gap in life expectancy of about 15 years for men and 10 years for women when comparing the most affluent 1% of individuals with the poorest 1%. In perspective, the 10-year life expectancy difference for women is equal to the decrement in longevity from a lifetime of smoking.”[325] As a measure of well-being, life expectancy has been influenced by many factors, but recently, increases have been mostly "driven by decreases in mortality at young age, but today, it is decreases in mortality at old age that increases life expectancy"[326] despite the higher levels of poverty that are also predominantly seen in the same two groups.

Even without the import of a 100-year pandemic, Kenya was already struggling with socio-economic development, expanding peoples’ opportunities, and overall, improving HDI indicators, even with the benefit of almost 60 years of independence. While one concedes that much progress has been made with HDI indices (life expectancy was 46 at independence, and has gone up to 68 today), Kenya is still classified as a lower middle-income country (LMIC) by the World Bank standards. Over a third of its population stills lives in poverty. Socio-economic development is being, and will be severely impacted by the pandemic for the foreseeable future. The government, now more than ever, needs more coherent strategies that go beyond the ‘Big Four’ pillars of development that the government of the day identified as the most important and immediate concerns.

As a matter of long-term planning, it is also important to examine the question of education, one of the most significant contributors to future human resources development, well-being (considering the relationship between education, heath, number of children and income potential) and an overall, better-educated populace that can advance a country’s lot. The simultaneous challenges of implementing a CBC curriculum and the pandemic’s negative effects portends long-term harm, and careful planning is needed, to ensure that learners are not unduly disadvantaged by the lost instruction time.

Considering early data that shows regression in learning and content acquisition, it is not enough to simply pick up where previous semesters left off. Educational authorities also need to consider the long-term effects of students who are out of school for long periods of time – up to six months in some instances – so as to mitigate the long term effects of being out of school for so long. It is inopportune to call for a reconsideration of the structure and

---

[325] Dave A. Chokshi, "Income, Poverty, and Health Inequality," *JAMA*, Vol. 319, No. 13 (2018): 1312-1313. doi:10.1001/jama.2018.252.

[326] Vladimir Canudas-Romo, "Life expectancy and poverty," *The Lancet - Global Health*, Vol. 6 (2018), e812, doi: https://doi.org/10.1016/S2214-109X(18)30327-9.

purposes of education at this point, but one considers it a future necessity – a reconsideration that does not just 'tweak' edges of a deeply flawed educational system that focuses on memorization of content, rather than on educating innovative job creators for a future that is full of climate change and unpredictable, hundred-year pandemics such as COVID-19.

Impact on Health, Care and Access

Kenya's health system leaves much to be desired. Even before COVID-19 became the albatross around most countries' health systems, the sight of Kenyans queueing outside hospitals for hours, being forced to travel miles and days to access healthcare services, inaccessible medicines or sale by hospitals even where they should be distributed for free, poor equipment, and other issues, were already exacting a price on the health of Kenyans. The National Hospital Insurance Fund (NHIF) works sporadically but is also rife with corruption and misuse, and more recently, subjected to 'raiding' by the rather well-compensated government employees. At the same time, elderly Kenyans are generally ineligible to be covered by health insurance, in itself a form of discrimination and terrible policy, for the elderly are more likely to be unwell and therefore, more likely to have health challenges and thus use health facilities at higher rates. COVID-19 then has the impact of diminishing their health and life expectancy.

One of the other anticipated impacts of the pandemic is the decrease in the utilization of health-care facilities even for treatment of other, non-COVID-19 diseases, out of fear that hospitals are good incubators and potential super-spreader locations, despite little evidence to support this suspicion. This leads to potential patients foregoing treatment, leading to public entreaties for citizens to continue using hospitals. Notwithstanding, government policy appears to regularly impose self-defeating conditions: for instance, the designation of COVID-19 hospitals decreased hospital utilization capacity. Considering that Kenya faces such other diseases such as Malaria, TB, HIV/AIDS, and measles,[327] in and of themselves also some of the major causes of deaths, the pandemic's impact thus continues to be severe. This is further complicated by the structure and mechanisms of financing healthcare

[327] Polet Njeri Ouma, Abednego Nzyuko Masai, and Israel Nyaburi Nyadera, "Health coverage and what Kenya can learn from the COVID-19 pandemic," *Journal of Global Health*, Vol. 10, No. 2 (2020): 020362. doi: 10.7189/jogh.10.020362.

in an age of reduced productivity, diminishing the overall ease and level of access and with it, the health of citizens.

Another complicating issue, rather outcome, of the pandemic, is the government's strategy that aims to decongest hospitals, including of those diagnosed with COVID-19, in favor of home treatment. While it is true that most individuals who contract COVID-19 do not end up in hospital, the existing levels of poverty, urban-to-rural migration and the nature of communal living (including multi-generational households often living in cramped spaces that do not lend themselves to social-distancing) can further complicate the health of the populace and allow for faster pandemic spread. Home treatment, without adequate monitoring by health authorities and just as often, without the proper equipment, can facilitate community contagion. This is because 'caring,' nurturing, is expected to be shown towards those experiencing poor health.

Kenyans recognize this paradox. On the one hand, home remedies and therapies have worked since time immemorial, but COVID-19 is also new. Further, there is a healthy amount of skepticism over whether or not COVID-19 even exists particularly given the way 'government' conducts itself. Popular 'myth' suggests that most doctors will not disclose a COVID-19 diagnosis even when one is suspected; that they have a step-up approach. If they suspect that a potential patient might be unable to handle news of a COVID-19 diagnosis and that they might likely to die of the news that they have COVID-19, rather than from the effects of the disease itself, it is labeled 'pneumonia.' The efficacy of home therapies is unclear.

Notwithstanding, the failure to modify various ceremonies and life in general continue(s) to facilitate transmission. A well-known radio personality, quoting the health CS, remarked sardonically, that 'individuals go to funeral and burial activities of COVID-19 victims, and the following week, they themselves are buried' having possibly contracted the virus at these events. Even without knowing if they have contracted COVID-19, Kenyans have taken to treating their perceived 'pneumonias' with home remedies, unknown if they actually work. However, this criticism may not be all unwarranted – in cases where hospitalization is not required even in western countries, managing positive diagnoses does frequently involve reduction of the symptom severity using some of the same local remedies that Kenyans have found to be useful, including lemon and ginger.

COVID-19 has sucked all the air from any discussions of most other diseases. It has led to a shift in focus, even by global compacts, private philanthropies and foundations that fund health and healthcare research.

Organizations such as the Bill and Melinda Gates Foundation, which previously focused their giving on innovations in WASH services, reproductive, maternal and infant health and mortality reduction, diseases and outbreaks such as cholera, Ebola and the Marburg fever, shifted most of their funding to COVID-19-related services.

In light of the previous discussion on the appreciable reticence of citizens to visit hospitals, COVID-19's indirect impact is that of keeping potential patients out of hospitals and away from care, further diminishing health outcomes. The almost irrational fear that going to hospital actually exposes the potential patient to COVID-19 and therefore, staying home with the non-COVID-19 illness, rather than seeking care, is a better option, will likely make the chronic conditions worse, or lead to alternative ways of dealing with maladies. This also applies to some of the vaccines that are necessary for the proper development of children. With the great consternation that is currently the focus of vaccines, other traditional, uncontested vaccines such as the polio and BCG have come under great scrutiny, and suspicion as to the timing and their objectives, in ways that citizens did not previously express. None of these potential outcomes are especially positive in the context of improving the overall health outcomes.

One potential silver lining to the whole pandemic is the marginal improvement in hygiene, as a result of the requirement to 'sanitize' and frequently wash hands, especially when entering the kinds of establishments that include food service, such as hotels and supermarkets. The contents of the sanitizing sprays are often suspect, looking and feeling more like ditch-water and soap, but on the whole, more people have taken to washing hands and generally improving their hygiene.

The infra-red no-contact thermometers that are used by many establishments are less predictable: they regularly show body temperatures of anywhere from 30°C to 38°C even absent contagion. They also occasionally fail to read the temperatures, suggesting that the whole enterprise is not useful. Further, measuring customer temperatures and then packing people like sardines inside supermarkets (as opposed to limiting the number of customers inside at any one time) demonstrates the self-defeating nature of the mitigation.

COVID-19's Impact on Mental Health

The COVID-19 pandemic has also lifted the curtain on another of the challenges that Kenyan society faces: the increasing, often unaddressed crisis of almost pandemic proportions, which is mental health. Mental health impacts have been hypothesized to manifest now and increase in the future. The WHO has found that currently, "stress and anxiety, and [...] a rise in depression, suicide and substance"[328] has been one of the early indicators. The future, it estimates, will be characterized by two peaks; "the first peak is dominated by anxiety and corresponds to the peak in COVID-19 cases. A second peak of negative mental health outcomes comprising of Post-Traumatic Stress Disorder (PTSD), depression, suicide, complicated grief bereavement, and relapse of those with existing disorders."[329]

Subsequent to the (hopefully near) end of the pandemic period, more of the latter is expected. But the realities of the situation in Kenya demonstrates that the appearance of both of these is not sequential. Although the country and the president have identified the need to focus on improving mental health, it takes some time to train practitioners who will then interface with the public, so as to assist with the public. A further challenge is encountered: this relates to attituded towards the issue of mental health, and the proposed cures (mostly, prayer). The lack of realization of diverse diagnoses that are possible with mental health, or strategies for mental wellness, further impede any progress.

During the duration of the pandemic, incidences of domestic violence that have led to murder, murder-suicides or other acts of extreme violence directed especially at women and girls, but to an increasingly greater extent, at entire families, have been on a rapid rise. Mental health is one of those issues that Kenyan society neglects, and when addressed, those persons experiencing the different diagnoses are quite often simply locked up and fed drugs to keep them near-comatose. Indeed, anyone finding themselves doing a stint at Mathare Hospital, and the hospital itself, is synonymous with being 'mad,' the all-encompassing description of any and all mental illnesses and diagnoses. 'Mad' people are treated very badly outside of hospital conditions, with evidence of being chained or spending most of their lives hidden from public view.

---

[328] Florence Jaguga and Edith Kwobah, "Mental health response to the COVID-19 pandemic in Kenya: a review," *International Journal of Mental Health Systems*, Vol. 14, No. 68 (2020). https://doi.org/10.1186/s13033-020-00400-8.

[329] Jaguga, "Mental health response to the COVID-19 pandemic," (2020).

'Madness' is used to label, or explain everything from schizophrenia to schizoaffective disorders, from bipolar disorders to depression: there is scant differentiation in the different mental diagnoses. But in the age of greater use of social media, of self-awareness and greater openness, increasingly, those affected are speaking publicly about their struggles. It would thus appear that mental illness is on the rise. This, taken together with the finding of "severe increases in maternal mental health issues, such as clinically relevant anxiety and depression"[330] among expectant women, the need becomes that much greater. What is clear is that the severity of mental illness requires the government to come up with a strategy for dealing with the issue, now (during the pandemic) and in the days to come, really, to ensure a healthy people.

On Government, Governance and Human Security

Security in the age of COVID-19 does not only imply protection from potential physical danger, but also from the very legal entity that abrogates to itself the obligation to enforce societal rules and regulations – the government. It is the same government that has monopoly over violence, that can legally kill one or more of its citizens, and in Kenya's case, has done so. Considering the pandemic's course, debates on security have often revolved around food security, given the diminished capacity to make a living on account of closures, lockdowns, travel bans and social distancing. The other discussion revolves around apps that carry out a variety of tasks related to COVID-19: monitor individuals' COVID-19 exposure, track and trace potentially infected persons, record and advise on exposure, and increasingly, to store 'COVID-19 passport' data, such as immunization status, and transmit that data to various other entities.[331]

Despite assurances that the government is not doing anything nefarious with the data, and the reality that the government potentially already has some, if not all of the data, paranoid citizens often consider government mandates on masks, vaccines, proposed vaccine passports and/or track and trace functions

---

[330] Bethany Kotlar, Emily Gerson, Sophia Petrillo, Ana Langer and Henning Tiemeier, "The impact of the COVID-19 pandemic on maternal and perinatal health: a scoping review," *Reproductive Health*, Vol.18, Nol. 10 (2021). https://doi.org/10.1186/s12978-021-01070-6.

[331] Surekha Borra, "COVID-19 Apps: Privacy and Security Concerns," In A. Joshi, N. Dey and K. Santosh, (eds), *Intelligent Systems and Methods to Combat Covid-19*, SpringerBriefs in Applied Sciences and Technology, Springer, (Singapore, 2020), https://doi.org/10.1007/978-981-15-6572-4_2.

unacceptable even though the stated goal is to assure general welfare within the shared polity. The position is informed by allegations that the government is possibly using the data to track citizens and thus violate their right to privacy, even though the right to privacy in Kenya is another of those weak, if not non-existent, institutional practices. A fair question, one whose proper answer and position will likely not be found in these pages, is where balance resides, between personal freedoms and privacy, versus need to protect the collective, public health lies, and what the government's role is.

For Kenya, another form of insecurity has manifested, since the very early days of the pandemic. This is the security of the person, and freedom from abuse by the government. March 27, 2020 remains an important day, considering how Kenyans were treated by NGAO officers enforcing curfew in Mombasa, fully two hours before curfew was scheduled to start. The goal, mission and reason for existence of the Kenya police is generally considered to include protection of the citizens, rather than murder them in the name of curfew. Human security conceived more broadly includes the security and autonomy of the person and that of their immediate environment. It thus demands that citizens' well-being should be guaranteed and human rights (and citizenship rights) guide mitigation actions. The COVID-19 cannot justify suspension of individuals' rights, including the right to be free from government coercion.

Because states and their ruling apparatus (governments) are established to ensure the welfare of the citizens, it is reasonable to expect that the state has an obligation to assure citizens of their security particularly when they consent to give up the right to private violence in dispute resolution. This has not been the general experience of the Kenyan citizen. Instances of police violence against citizens are well and widely chronicled. The police (broadly, representing and functioning as an arm of government) has been squarely in the limelight over the killing of two brothers in Embu recently, ostensibly, while enforcing curfew, in addition to the more than 20 other citizens killed during curfew enforcement since March 2020.[332] It is really scandalous that citizens can be killed for no reason other than being late and thus violated curfew – this speaks to the value police attach to citizens' lives.

Human security ought to include freedom from violence (state-level) and at the personal level, any domestic, gender and intimate partner violence, the latter especially deterred through concerted actions and taking violence

[332] Abdi Latif Dahir, "Deaths in custody of two brothers fuel anger over Covid enforcement in Kenya," *New York Times - Coronavirus Updates*, Aug. 16, 2021, https://www.nytimes.com/2021/08/16/world/africa/kenya-covid-enforcement-brothers-death.html.

seriously, rather than as 'something that is in the domain of the home.' The government should account for and ensure the well-being of the girl child, of women and vulnerable groups in society. Human security demands that citizens be protected from oppression including by the government, and when it is unable to do that, mechanisms exist to ensure that it does – hence the ICC. This is the next task that faces the Kenyan government, to insure the level of human security. It is one at which the Kenyan government has not excelled. The country needs to uphold its end of the contract with its citizens, to assure their well-being. The state would also do well to end, and punish culprits of the state-sponsored terror that has been visited upon citizens in the name of COVID-19.

Government functionaries, its agents and more generally, elites' record of obeying directives that the self-same issues to citizens is very poor. As the pandemic infects, even continues to kill more and more people, the government continues to send mixed signals regarding the enforcement of lockdowns, bans and curfews. It often appears that the government is following the mantra that suggests 'do what I say, not what I do' and as such, public political rallies, whether to tout the Building Bridges Initiative (BBI) or the celebration of national holidays, these are all potential contagion points and channels for diseases and vectors. Banning public rallies and then going ahead to hold one, whether it is presented in the form of 'harambee' or 'inspecting development projects', or 'national holiday celebration,' it is clear that the government has not committed itself to ensuring the success of its own directives. Perhaps the 2022 election is driving some of this reticence and continued meetings, but one ought to remember that SARS-CoV-2 is no respecter of elections. Or BBI. Or personal freedoms.

One of the other areas that the government has failed to address is that of business. According to some recent estimates, including from the Central Bank of Kenya, business losses stemming from the pandemic are running at about 20%.[333] Granted, agriculture accounts for a significant portion of the GDP and the profitable employment of Kenyan citizens. However, if 20% of businesses have become casualties of the pandemic, the government ought to consider strategies to shore up such businesses, including the provision of financial facilities and support to keep them running. Businesses also provide employment, and their collapse implies decreased levels of employment and therewith, a loss of PAYE and purchasing power. In fact, businesses in Kenya

[333] Victor Amadala, "Corona has wiped out 20% of small businesses — CBK report," *MSN*, 27/07/2021, URL: https://www.msn.com/en-xl/africa/kenya/corona-has-wiped-out-20-of-small-businesses-cbk-report/ar-AAMARI8?li=BB12Iwuk.

are tied to many other sectors, including transport. Stories of private schools-turned-chicken-breeders have abounded; it is clear that government's lack of strategies to shore up businesses, or assist them to recover, has immediate, but also long-term negative impacts on the economic outlook whenever the country begins to recover from the pandemic.

COVID-19's Law(s) of Dynamic Negatives

Perhaps it is inevitable, that every new process begets the opportunity for rent-seeking, corruption and fraud at every level of society in countries like Kenya. If Al Capone could find ways to circumvent the Prohibition by bootlegging liquor all over the US and getting wealthy off of some illegal venture, and long before him, 'entrepreneurs' who sold the so-called 'indulgences' – devices intended to 'purchase' individuals out of 'purgatory,' Kenyans officials at all levels of government demonstrated perfect capability and willingness to profit from the imposition of new rules and mandates. Already, the country was on everyone's 'worst-case' list – the World Bank, Transparency International, Paris Club of Donors, failed states index – thus any credible lender and donor exhibits a healthy skepticism over Kenya's governance record and structures.

When seat-belts were introduced in *matatus* in 2004, Kenyans were unenthusiastic in using, or embracing them, even though their ultimate goal was to save passengers' lives. The Kenya traffic police roadblocks became the venue for 'sanctioning' passengers. Most of the time, the officers imposed instant 'fines,' which the Kenyan government is very unlikely to have either received or benefited from. In the more recent past, the government's procurement processes became the new cash cow: supplying air in place of goods, sub-standard goods and over-inflating the supplied items. One of the most laughable, and ridiculously overpriced instances of rent-seeking was the $1,028 per unit of wheelbarrows that were purchased in Bungoma County in 2015.[334] Investigations, even when they are commissioned, rarely snag culprits, or the said accused use the court processes to prolong the legal proceedings so that even 30 years after the Goldenberg 'hot air-gold' export scandal first came to light, no satisfactory conclusion has ever been reached in

334 Maureen Murimi, "Bungoma residents protest Ksh 100,000 wheelbarrows," *Citizen Digital*, Updated September 8, 2015, https://citizentv.co.ke/news/bungoma-residents-protest-ksh-100000-wheelbarrows-100195/.

the matter, and the accused roam the country free. Such is the state of governance.

COVID-19 moved the ‘connected’ Kenyans from the longer-term ‘tenderpreneurs’ and into the better-resourced ‘COVID millionaires.’ This really just shifted the source of illicit money from the long-term government tenders to the more easily obtainable COVID-19 funds. The shift was facilitated by the urgent nature of the COVID-19 pandemic and the need to procure and distribute resources such as PPE that would help the country test, trace and protect citizens and thus reduce transmission. Even in a time of need, where citizens actually faced ruin from a rapidly-spreading pandemic, the opportunity to find ways to short-change government, citizens, donors and literally, everyone involved in the process, was one of the more unbelievable outcomes of the pandemic in Kenya. Despite the shift from the old ‘tenderpreneurship,’ the underlying structures of high-level corruption and petty graft were left intact. At the pedestrian level, one surmises that *especially* the police stumbled into more avenues of corruption.

The new avenues included police enforcement of masks mandates, policing (or profiting from) adherence to curfews, letting especially hospitality businesses, bars and clubs continue operating for a fee, so long as the doors are closed to give the appearance of the curfew being in effect. That even pandemic mitigation can become a source of personal enrichment speaks to an entrenched culture of corruption at such high levels that the country is essentially a bandit nation. Additional ‘creativity’ seen in enforcing the mandates has further imperiled the broader global community. For instance, although the government requires a negative, COVID-19 test before anyone can fly out of the country, reports regularly emerge that show that some do leave the country without the requisite test. Naturally, there is often a greasing of palms, with substitutions of trusted traveler codes so that one can board the flight. One surmises that the possibility of future variants of COVID-19 could be transmitted that way.

Problems with the overall enforcement of COVID-19 mitigation strategies denotes the classic case of individuals working against their best interests. Whereas many other countries other than Kenya – including more isolated island nations such as Australia with less porous borders – have failed to contain the rise, or spread, of new variants or COVID-19 as a whole, the attitudes demonstrated by especially health officials and particularly law enforcement is troubling. No one can know which variants will take root, or who will be infected by COVID-19 as a result of the actions taken by immigration officials, police officers, port health officers and others tasked with enforcing quarantines and assuring that travelers have negative COVID-19 tests. The nature of short-term gains that such officials pursue, at the expense of a broader, birds-eye-view of the necessity of containing the pandemic, is almost tragic.

This brings us to another issue, one that is perhaps uniquely Kenyan: fatalistic, fantastic, even magical thinking and attitudes towards the pandemic and life. Granted, no one can control much of what happens in the broader realm of life though individuals have and exercise the capacity to make decisions. However, the notion that 'the graph is drawn,' often expressed as 'inshallah,' or 'Ngai enda,' suggests that man has no capacity to affect the future, and that if one will die of COVID-19, then there is nothing one could possibly do to change this reality, this future, notwithstanding *The Adjustment Bureau* and potential to change one's destiny. As such, the notion that if one will die of COVID-19, nothing under the sun can change that outcome leads to reckless health behaviors even at the risk of infecting others, particularly given the breakthrough version of the pandemic.

A different variation of the *inshallah* philosophy is the notion of 'curses.' In more recent literature and in the African context, these refer to natural resources and the tensions they induce.[335] In the more traditional meaning, a 'curse' is interchangeably used with 'witchcraft,' 'spiritual evil' and are generally seen as "a means of explaining the unequal distribution of good and bad fortune, and the occurrence of otherwise inexplicable misfortune."[336] Evidently, COVID-19 is one such evil. In some communities, those diagnosed with COVID-19 have been subjected to different attempts at being 'cleansed' of such curses, such evil. To disabuse one of the notion that COVID-19 is not induced by witchcraft or evil spirits, and that its transmission is accomplished in the normal course of daily activities can be a challenge, perhaps illustrating and explaining part of the difficulty the Kenyan government faces getting some elements of its society to take the pandemic seriously, or the elimination of those communal practices designed to 'cure' witchcraft, which may in instances further exacerbate the likelihood of increased transmission.

These attitudes are also expressed by phrases that translate into, 'no one will die all (the whole) day,' suggesting that if COVID-19 does indeed kill an

---

[335] Artwell Nhemachena, Nelson Mlambo and Maria Kaundjua, "The Notion of the "Field" and the Practices of Researching and Writing Africa: Towards Decolonial Praxis," *Africology: The Journal of Pan African Studies*, vol. 9, no. 7, (September 2016), 15-36.

[336] Jean La Fontaine, "Witchcraft belief is a curse on Africa," The Guardian - Africa Comment, 1st March, 2012, https://www.theguardian.com/commentisfree/belief/2012/mar/01/witchcraft-curse-africa-kristy-bamu.

individual, it won't be an all-day affair (this is not necessarily true, and the suffering has often been described as horrendous). Such fatalistic attitudes are totally unhelpful in the attempts at controlling the pandemic, especially coupled with vaccine hesitancy. Other related attitudes are captured in some of the community beliefs and sayings; for instance: '*gũtirĩ wa Gĩkũyũ ũkuuaga atarogetwo'* (no one among the Kikuyu dies without the death being attributed to 'witchcraft'). This is an unfortunate, double-edged sword, the implication, perhaps well-deserved, is that for anyone who dies during the duration of the pandemic, the death is likely to be attributed to COVID-19 even if it is not. Such unhelpful attitudes make it less likely for especially the skeptical and traditionalist community members to take the pandemic seriously.

Alongside the fatalistic attitude, skepticism regarding the existence of COVID-19 is also quite widespread. It is a perspective supported by some of the government's own actions. It is partly fed by general distrust of government and the perception that it is corrupt, seeking for some advantage over the citizen to benefit especially elites. It contributes to the perceived minimization of the potential impact of the pandemic to citizens. Theoretically, if COVID-19 existed, the thinking goes, the government would take seriously the implementation of the measures it announces periodically. For many Kenyans, COVID-19 is also dismissed as one of the many 'flus' that have manifested. And, so the belief goes, 'no one ever died of the flu.'

It is the case that COVID-19 is a form of influenza, one that is decidedly more contagious and that has no known cure to date. As such, dismissing COVID-19 as one type of 'flu' risks not taking it seriously, paying attention to the pandemic mitigation strategies and potentially, making its impact even worse. But even more importantly, considering that the government has made few periodic, perfunctory, statements to debunk myths such as that COVID-19 vaccines cause infertility, or people to grow bigger on one side than the other. Public education and sensitization are only used to the extent that government is increasing or lifting some containment measures, and almost all of its actions are largely punitive. Thus, the combined impacts of the pandemic are likely to continue negatively affecting the country for the foreseeable future, and the persistent myths and beliefs around COVID-19 and vaccines persist.

To reinvent the wheel when one already exists can be unnecessary. Learning from others' mistakes is s more strategic approach than learning all the lessons. The US's (and to some extent, the UK's) response to the pandemic, in the early months of 2020, was a study in some of what *not* to do. Skepticism, proposing bad science and bad cures, the government's inability to provide consistent and evidence-based guidance, the privileging of politics over science, the economy over survival, are now well etched into the world's consciousness.

Kenya's path out of the pandemic requires the government and citizens to prioritize science over socio-political, socio-cultural and to some extent, economic actions and preferences. True, ceremonies such as burials, weddings and bride-price are part of the human experience, but they are conducted on the backs of rapid increases in the number of COVID-19 infections, hospitalizations and deaths. Basic survival ought to dictate that the festivals, celebrations and political rallies should be shelved until it is safe to hold them again. There might eventually be a need for practices such as pouring libations and other cultural compensatory strategies, but the number of fatalities will have been significantly reduced. After all, there cannot be culture if there are no people to practice it.

Amid the new phenomenon of ‘vaccine nationalism’ and the hoarding until expiry of vaccines that western nations often don’t need and do not use, African countries, Kenya included, have sought to find alternatives to current strategies of depending on (scant) western nations’ largesse for access to vaccines. The global recognition that African nations, and most lower income and lower-to-middle income countries currently do not have the capacity to avail themselves of vaccines, coupled with the intellectual property-driven western nations, has led to the alternative of COVAX, the COVID-19 Vaccines Global Access program designed to close the gap. COVAX is encompasses GAVI, CEPI and WHO, comported by the EU and the French government, and previously leveraged India’s global pharmaceutical manufacturing capacity to fulfil its pledges to Africa and other nations for vaccines. However, as of September 2021, most of Kenya’s vaccines come from well-wishers and donor nations such as Greece, the US and Latvia.

It bears repeating, that while testing 2.5 million Kenyans over a period of 550 days (so far) is a decent achievement, but a woefully inadequate one, considering the seroprevalence tests. Results that show X number of positive cases out of Y samples, giving Z positivity rates, touted almost daily on TV, are misleading at least, and at worst, deceptive, lulling citizens into a false sense of security. Increasing testing would be especially welcome, but perhaps shifting focus to seroprevalence would give health authorities a better sense of community spread. It might also help determine the level of contagion and how well individuals are coping, especially if they have been previously infected and recovered, assess the state of antibodies formation and therewith, alternative approaches to managing the pandemic. As things stand now, even the government cannot exactly fathom how widespread the pandemic is. Were it to be established that it has already swept through most of the population, alternative management strategies might be considered and implemented.

During the course of the pandemic, Madagascar came in for much derision, on account of the idea that there were traditional herbal cures for the pandemic (coupled with prayers). Whereas there has been little by way of assessment of the efficacy of the traditional cures, one cannot necessarily dismiss them out of hand. Traditional cures have been used for as long as man has been around, and some do have benefits (even if it's such compounds as THC). Kenyans have used a variety of combination concoctions that include ginger, lemon, (boiled) blue gum tree leaves, *Wanjirũ wa rũrii, mũnua nũgũ, mu-arubaini* (Neem tree), *mũceege,* among other compounds, have been thought to alleviate symptoms of pneumonia, cold, flu and some suspect, even COVID-19. Dismissing the potential efficacy of these cures is potential folly; after all, most of medications derive from the self-same plants and trees and traditional knowledge has in the past been known to hold value.

Other Miscellaneous Impacts and Proposals for Effectiveness

There are a myriad of other issues that have issued from the pandemic, some that expose the level of preparation (or not) of various sectors of the Kenyan economy and government with regard to efficient management of issues within and without. When COVID-19 struck, many governments imposed travel bans and Kenya was among them. Besides the debacle of quarantines that the government flubbed, the implementation of the curfews and other related issues, the problem of Kenyans stranded abroad, and reports of their mistreatment became a most significant challenge. This was especially the case with Kenyans in China and in the Arab and Gulf States, with limited consular support by the government, and extended to the working hours of consulates and embassies to provide documentation so as to facilitate travel to Kenya especially as the lockdowns persisted.

Simultaneously, there are silver linings even within the context of the pandemic. Although Kenya's COVID-19 numbers are quite suspect, considering those countries that have managed to rein in the pandemic by way of vaccinations, there exists opportunities for gradual, safe reopening of the economy and bringing back some of the tourist dollars that would boost the livelihoods and herald some return to normalcy. Of course, this would require verification of vaccinations and ensuring that best health and hygiene practices can be sustained. Rather than engage in what appears to be retaliation – for instance, banning flights to the UK and Tanzania in retaliation thereof – and considering the 'pent-up demand' that tourists are seen to harbor, it is useful to consider scalpels, rather than machetes, to safely begin the gradual reopening of the economy. One might suggest that 'Europeans and Americans are vaccinated, frustrated and eager to escape wildfires, heat domes, heat waves and are eager to see a bit of wildlife,' thus are a ripe tourist market.

On the political front, the Kenyan government and especially elites, refuse to act as if COVID-19 exists, or is lethal. Sporadic, unenforced bans on meetings and political activity continues to both undercut the government's rules, and requests that citizens implement strategies to help contain pandemic. Citizens can be forgiven for doubting the seriousness of the pandemic, or its existence. If COVID-19 existed, would government ban public political gatherings, but then go ahead and hold national celebrations such as the Madaraka Day festivities in Kisumu in June 2021, with scant adherence to COVID-19 mitigation strategies?

More importantly, government actions lead to a serious erosion of credibility and authority on its, a decidedly dangerous outcome. The skepticism about COVID-19 has gradually morphed into a distrust of most things government says and does, especially vaccines. There are allegations that the vaccines are filled with water, that the president would never have allowed himself to be injected with an experimental medical 'compound,' particularly if it does, as alleged, lead to infertility and being fat on one side of the recipient's body. Government communications strategy fails to counter these types of rumors and misinformation that characterizes debates about the pandemic, the mitigation strategies and even vaccines, to the detriment of the country and the likelihood of containing the pandemic and returning the country to pre-pandemic, or other near 'normal' reality.

Along with the concerns regarding public meetings, the government's July 2021 decision to end the social distancing measures in the public transport sector, especially after modifications to matatus to account for social-distancing was confounding, and quite widely panned. It has often been described, derisively, as 'the government has decided that poor people should die.' It is likely that the government recognized that social-distancing in matatus, while cramming all other venues, including super-markets or matatu queues, defeated the original purpose. Yet the decision can only compound the challenges that COVID-19 entails. Further, if there is no social distancing in the transport sector, does it make any sense to continue enforcing such measures as curfews? After all, hotels and bars are likely to be less crowded than matatus and buses – again, this is an element of interesting government reversals without taking into account the entire spectrum of the implications of the decisions.

The decision, coming as the delta variant was sweeping Kenya and the overall positivity rate climbing, hospitalization accelerating and the debacle of India's experience with the variant still fresh, and with vaccines remaining as close as a space program project, it is clear government decisions do not inspire confidence or sentiment that it is especially competent, willing or able to contain COVID-19. Then again, it has only been 550 days since the first case. Perhaps there is a grand strategy hiding in the coffers of the Ministry of Health or Harambee House. But given other items of trust that Kenyan citizens have been asked to bestow on the government – eradicating corruption, ensuring security, providing for their general welfare – this seems like a bet whose outcome is iffy.

There are short-term plans and programs to consider, as well as long-term disaster preparedness to consider, not only for Kenya, but for the entire planet. Kenya has scientists, and facilities that have done some work with pandemics and viruses (including sequencing COVID-19 variants); it can leverage that capacity, individually and together with other organizations such as the WHO and Africa CDC, GSK and other health and wellness organizations so as to resolve this, and future pandemics. After all, most of the predictions suggest that animal-to-human virus contagion will increase in future, not decrease. It thus behooves Africa to come up with a moon-shot program that will assist member states to meet the health challenges – current and future – with and without the rest of the world if necessary.

Conclusion

An Overview of the State of Affairs: February 2020 – February 2022

The foregoing has illuminated the opening moments of SARS-CoV-2, the virus that would become COVID-19, as it began making the rounds around the world in November through January 2020. It has chronicled the rise of new vocabulary, a new way of life – essentially, creating an age and experience 'before COVID-19', and 'during COVID-19', more popularly referred to as the 'new normal.' One hopes that there will be an 'after COVID-19', although current optimistic projections suggest that the virus is transitioning from a pandemic to an endemic stage. Perhaps this is the case; foretelling the future is essentially a perilous affair. And so, the question does issue: can one accurately analyze the progress, developments and possible outlook of the future of the pandemic, and how Kenya will eventually look like at the end – if there is an end – to and of the pandemic? Having incomplete knowledge is no reason to not attempt such an undertaking, even though one concedes that a future volume will probably issue.

There is potential peril, but also promise of learned lessons, in considering in a wholesome manner, Kenya's handling of the COVID-19 pandemic. This is because of the very nature of the pandemic itself. Around the winter months of 2020, as the first vaccines against the COVID-19 pandemic were coming online, there was almost palpable hope that finally, the world would nail the very efficient, very persistent virus. *Then came the Delta variant.* It was arguably a horror show out of India, with the funeral pyres burning day and night, bodies dumped into the Ganges, and heartbreaking pictures of families desperately running helter-skelter to try and find oxygen. Soon, as summer approached, it appeared that the worst was behind the country.

But as has so often happened with COVID-19, the Delta variant soon became the overwhelmingly transmissible variant, crowding out most of the other previous variants. It was more contagious, arguably more deadly, and more concerning. Most people, by now having been home for more than a year, working, learning, teaching from home and avoiding every facet of social life, were ready for an end to masks and restrictions. Western nations and their capitals became the battlefield for freedom versus occupying most political debates. Even in Kenya, the extended, seemingly never-ending curfews and lockdowns caused a lot of chafing. In response, the Kenyan government varied the lockdowns, targeting the curfews to those counties that were experiencing high infection, case numbers and positivity rates.

The more unexpected development was perhaps not the discovery of a new variant (Omicron) after humanity believed that we had seen the worst of the pandemic: it was the ferocity with which the Omicron variant exploded, infecting within three to six short months, the same number of people as all the other variants had in almost eighteen months. Suddenly, everything we had known about the pandemic changed. The prospect of reopening previously locked-down communities looked bleak. A collective groan was heard, and a resumption of WFH and all its attendant crises became like a looping repeat. There is no knowing when, where and how COVID-19 will come to a conclusion, or what lives and communities will look like. Whether or not people will return to offices full time, or whether we will have discovered that physical interaction can be a pathway to pandemic blues, is yet to be clear.

Still, we must take stock of the past two years (as of February 2022), and in Kenya's case, the past 600 days, and everything that has transpired in the interim. It is useful to remind readers that although some countries have seen a fifth wave of the pandemic (Omicron in the US was more like a fourth wave), Kenya has been experiencing a surge in Omicron cases in what is considered a *fifth* wave. This is likely to be exacerbated by the start of a campaign season leading up to the 2022 general elections in August. It is still unclear how campaigning in a fifth pandemic wave will look, or what it will produce, but one suspects it is not going to be a positive outcome.

This Volume: Reviewing Kenya's Situation to 600 Days

The stated objective of this volume is to consider Kenya's responses and reactions to the pandemic, at the level of the government and society. As a complex society, straddling elements of modernity and socio-cultural, historical and religious realities, its responses have been nothing but fascinating, and suspiciously, a little too closely fashioned after those of the United Kingdom. It was thus necessary to not only begin by examining the timeline of the COVID-19 pandemic in Kenya, but to also examine the particular and select key figures, offices, groups, bureaucracies and organizations that have been most visible in managing the pandemic, from the Cabinet Secretary (the title fashioned after the US) in the Ministry of Health (fashioned after the UK), and their success or lack thereof.

An assessment of government administrative responses and strategies has demonstrated that, while the government did a decent job of communicating through near-daily press conferences, while signaling good practices (from hand sanitizing to wearing masks to avoiding handshakes), there was a gap between what the government's NERC committee was doing and saying, and what was being witnessed all over the country. Elites and politicians made a habit of addressing 'non-political' gatherings couched as 'meet-the-people-tours', 'prayer meetings' or 'inspecting development projects.' It has been an unconvincing, transparently deceptive strategy, and the leaders have been unable to assure that at such gatherings, their supporters were following good and proper hygiene and mitigation strategies.

Early in the pandemic, the government moved quickly and aggressively to attempt to contain the pandemic – almost impossible, unless you are an island nation like Madagascar or New Zealand – but also imposed rather draconian measures where alternatives were less than feasible. The closure of educational institutions, for example, did not just deprive pupils of education (the whole premise of online learning is as practical and viable as finding a live, breathing dinosaur) in a land of internet-by-megabyte, more outage than power (power outages), vanishingly few trained IT teachers and even ELE-rare computers for teachers to use. But pupils in almost half the counties in Kenya got school lunch in school, and without any delivery or pick-up systems as we have seen in the west, that was another marker for hunger and malnutrition. The physical assault of 'curfew violators,' a full two hours before curfew kicked in, demonstrated not only human rights violations, but also the expected future conduct of public safety officials.

The epidemiological responses that were proposed, *nee,* imposed, were sound. However, to ask Kenyans to purchase KN-95 masks, or get vaccinated before they could access government services sounded like a harebrained idea. The notion that people could sanitize – in a country with little by way of running water – was almost laughable. The level to which the sanitizing agents were diluted rendered them useless. Masks, initially allowing any variety including bandannas, shawls, scarfs and a host of similar coverings, were gradually adopted, but little clarification was given on how long they could be used. One was wont to find a simple surgical mask being used for a week, *continuously*, with nary a moment to even wash them. Where and when school resumed, most children had 5 surgical masks, one for each day. The question of whether masks have been worn for show is a valid one, particularly as newer and more aggressive variants issue.

Asking Kenyans about the most salient and most memorable elements of the COVID-19 pandemic might produce a simple answer: 'COVID-19 Millionaires.' That billions of shillings were provided to the country by the World Bank, in order to help mitigate the effects of COVID-19, and that most of it was embezzled, is not necessarily surprising to Kenyans. *Of course* we expected it. It is what government does. Perhaps at this point we should begin to wonder, what's wrong with whoever is at the World Bank (or other donor countries and agencies); do they not know that any assistance that goes through the government *will* be embezzled, as sure as the sun will rise the next day? One must conclude that whoever doles out the money is instructed, under pain of death, to give away the money. *No, World Bank, little of your money went to actually help Kenyans mitigate the pandemic.* And so we hope it was not a loan, just your bad money.

During the pandemic, Kenyans' 'peculiar' habits returned: this time, to masks. Whether it was the practice of sharing masks at the sign of police, wearing the mask on the chin, washing a surgical mask until it shed all the blue, crafting new, one-layer, surgical-looking-mask and a host of other poor habits, the pandemic offered opportunities for police officers to practice petty corruption. After all, one could expect that the 'big fish' were eating and the small fish, which were literally in the middle of the rich pickings, ought to eat too. It is absolutely tragic that even as it became clear that the KEMSA debacle was a *bona fide* scandal, the subsequent *circus* and lack of prosecutions continue to show what Kenya is – famously, *nchi ya kitu kidogo.* If anyone expects that any prosecutions will come out of that *charade,* they have another think coming.

Quarantine turned out to be one of the worst ideas in Kenya, essentially primed to either produce corruption or escape. No one in their right mind would have paid US$100 per day to stay at a hostel in KU or KMTC. One could literally stay at a decent downtown hotel, with breakfast and TV, for US$22 a night. What was tragic was that even after the suicide of a young South African in quarantine, the facilities did not get better. It actually made sense – as terrible as this sounds – that anyone caught in the trap of not having a mask, or eventually, wearing a *chin mask*, would attempt to get out of the proceedings as fast as they could. After all, if a two-week period in quarantine would result in a charge of US$1,400 – roughly about the amount of money a Kenyan will make in one year – escape was *the* only plausible strategy.

There are many puzzles surrounding Kenya's whole COVID-19 strategy, and although one would not endeavor towards conspiracy theory, they are head-scratchers. Everywhere, testing has been one of the most critical avenues to determining how widespread the pandemic is. Yet Kenya's testing regime is probably one of the weakest anywhere on the continent of Africa, perhaps except for Somalia, without a government. For most of the pandemic, Kenya generally never tested more than 10,000 people on any given day. As such, it has recorded a measly 3 million+ tests. There is no knowing how many of those are repeat tests (for example, this author has taken at least 3 during trips and entry/departure). It is likely then, that the single individuals tested are far fewer than 3 million. But there might be a strategy there. The fewer tests you do, the fewer you are likely to report as positive. Even if one reported that 10,000 people tested positive, it is still less terrifying than the 1.4 million one-day cases the US reported at the height of Omicron.

Just like most other countries, Kenya experienced, for a significant period of time, great vaccine hesitancy, misinformation, ridiculous assertions and outright lies as to what was in the vaccine and what it did to the body. That said, considering that almost 15.5 million shots have been administered as of February 2022, the hesitancy is less than one might expect. The Kenyan government, even as it was making the vaccines available, did not quite succeed in publicizing the vaccines as safe, available, and beneficial to the public. Similarly, actively debunking the widely-debunked myths, that Bill Gates somehow tracks individuals through the vaccine or other similar unbelievable rumors is important. This is, and ought to be good use of public information campaigns and widely available media.

There are other equally important issues that have been exposed by COVID-19, whether it is the lack of a social safety net, poor planning strategies (for example, designating some of the biggest and best-equipped hospitals as COVID-19 units), requiring businesses to shut down their operations and schools to discontinue instruction among other controls demonstrated some level of haphazard decision-making. In particular, some of this was done – such as imposing lockdowns – without providing alternative sources of support, which inevitably led to the need to violate the said restrictions, if one wanted to eat. It was not clear that there was a sound analysis of how the lockdowns would impact the populace, particularly considering the levels of poverty that persist in the country. There was a higher probability of dying from starvation than from catching COVID-19, and one hopes that the government was cognizant of these realities.

The pandemic has had a gendered dimension to it, and it would be unfortunate to ignore this dimension. As 'expected' caregivers, a most discriminatory prospect, women in Kenya have shouldered much of the burden of taking care of those who catch the virus. At the same time, the overall level of hardship imposed by the pandemic has seen women subjected to increasing levels of intimate partner violence (IPV) and gender-based crimes, from teenage pregnancies to rape and related negative experiences. Given the socio-cultural approach that government often takes to these issues, it is clear that dismissing them as 'domestic issues' is insufficient, and that more needs to be done especially to provide care and assistance, destigmatize and support mental health wellness, so that the frequent homicides and overall violence towards women will decrease. It should also address the rise of once defunct cultural practices, such as female circumcision and Female Genital Mutilation (FGM) which have been on the increase during the pandemic.

COVID-19 is no reason for the violation of Kenyans' civil and human rights. Managing the pandemic must not violate Kenyans' rights, particularly in such callous and needless ways as the Likoni Ferry whippings that were witnessed on the first day of the curfew, or with the killing of the two brothers in Embu – although this is often considered more of a theft situation. But human security goes beyond not being arbitrarily whipped or arrested by the police. It is also connected to availability of and food security, to ensure nutrition and wellness, and more broadly, ensure human development, access to health and healthcare and related matters. One might expand this all the way to ensuring better government and governance, in order to not only survive the pandemic, but to also thrive, whenever the curtain comes down on the pandemic.

The final chapter on COVID-19 is yet to be written, and may not be written for a little while. However, we have observed, throughout the past two years or thereabouts, that mankind learns, adapts, changes, and survives. Kenya has learnt, adapted, changed and survived, and at some point, going beyond survival to thriving is necessary and desirable. The past 600 days have challenged Kenya, but one hopes in the coming days and months, Kenya will have learnt lessons that address issues such as virtual working, fully online access to government services, alternative educational content delivery, and more importantly, fire-proofing systems so that they are ready for the next hundred-year pandemic, or whatever pandemic might be in the works.

References

_____ 2013. "*Incidence and Complications of Unsafe Abortion in Kenya: Key Findings of a National Study*." Nairobi: African Population and Health Research Center, MoH Kenya, IPAS, and Guttmacher Institute.

AA.com. 2020. "COVID-19: Kenya bans political rallies, extends curfew." *Anadolu Agency – Africa, Latest on Coronavirus outbreak.* Accessed April 11th, 2021. https://www.aa.com.tr/en/africa/covid-19-kenya-bans-political-rallies-extends-curfew/2032358#.

AAFP. 2021. "CDC Releases Interim Flu Vaccine Effectiveness Report." *The American Academy of Family Physicians.* Accessed 12th July 2021. https://www.aafp.org/news/health-of-the-public/20200226interimfluve.html.

Abbas, Muhammad Zaheer. 2020. "Practical implications of 'vaccine nationalism:' A short-sighted and risky approach in response to COVID-19." *Research Paper No. 124.* South Centre, Geneva.

Abdalla, Safa, Elizabeth G Katz, and Gary L Darmstadt. 2021. "Gender and the impact of COVID-19 on demand for and access to health care: analysis of data from Kenya, Nigeria, and South Africa." *The Lancet – Global Health – Special Issue*, Vol. 9, No., S7. Accessed July 20, 2021. doi: https://doi.org/10.1016/S2214-109X(21)00115-7.

Abdullahi, Leila, et al. 2020. "Community interventions in Low—And Middle-Income Countries to inform COVID-19 control implementation decisions in Kenya: A rapid systematic review." *PLOS One.* Accessed June 15th, 2021 https://doi.org/10.1371/journal.pone.0242403.

Adetifa, Ifedayo M.O. et al. 2021. "Temporal trends of SARS-CoV-2 seroprevalence in transfusion blood donors during the first wave of the COVID-19 epidemic in Kenya," *medRxiv.* Accessed July 20, 2021. doi: https://doi.org/10.1101/2021.02.09.21251404.

Africa CDC. "Coronavirus Disease 2019 (COVID-19) – Africa CDC COVID-19 Dashboard." *Africa Centres for Disease Control and Prevention (Africa CDC*), July 16th, 2021, https://africacdc.org/covid-19/.

Africa Center for Strategic Studies. 2020. "Lessons from the 1918-1919 Spanish Flu Pandemic in Africa," *Africa Center for Strategic Studies.* Accessed May 13th, 2021. https://africacenter.org/spotlight/lessons-1918-1919-spanish-flu-africa/.

Aloui-Zarrouk Z, L et al. 2020. "The wearing of face masks in African countries under the COVID 19 crisis: luxury or necessity?" *AAS Open Research* Vol. 2. Accessed July 20, 2021. https://doi.org/10.12688/aasopenres.13079.1.

Alwala, Bernard. 2020. "What Has Science to Do with Religion? A Looming Challenge of Traditional and Religious Practices on Curbing the Spread of COVID-19 Pandemic in

Kenya." *East African Journal of Traditions, Culture and Religion*, Vol. 2, No. 1: 22-33 Accessed May 20th, 2021. doi: https://doi.org/10.37284/2707-5370.

Amoth, Patrick. N.D. "Interim Guidelines on Management of COVID-19 in Kenya: COVID-19, Infection Prevention and Control (IPC) and Case Management." *Ministry of Health, Republic of Kenya.* https://kma.co.ke/Documents/Case%20management%20protocol.pdf.

Andam, Kwaw S., Hyacinth Edeh, Victor Oboh, Karl Pauw, and James Thurlow. 2020. *Estimating the economic costs of COVID-19 in Nigeria.* Lagos: IFPRI Nigeria.

Aragie, Emerta, Xinshen Diao, Sherman Robinson, Gracie Rosenbach, David J. Spielman, and James Thurlow. 2021. *Assessing the economywide impacts of COVID-19 on Rwanda's economy, agri-food system, and poverty.* Strategy Support Program/WP 01. Kigali: IFPRI Rwanda.

Austrian, Karen, et al. 2021. "Gendered economic, social and health effects of the COVID-19 pandemic and mitigation policies in Kenya: evidence from a prospective cohort survey in Nairobi informal settlements." *British Medical Journal (BMJ) Open*. doi: 10.1136/bmjopen-2020-042749. Accessed April 28, 2021.

Bai, Nina. 2020. "Still Confused About Masks? Here's the Science Behind How Face Masks Prevent Coronavirus." *Patient Care – University of California San Francisco*. Accessed September 26, 2021 https://www.ucsf.edu/news/2020/06/417906/still-confused-about-masks-heres-science-behind-how-face-masks-prevent.

Baicus, Anda. 2012. "History of polio vaccination." *World Journal of Virology* vol. 12; No. 1 (4): 108–114. Accessed July 20, 2021. doi: 10.5501/wjv.v1.i4.108.

Banga, Karismha and Dirk Willem te Velde. 2020. "COVID-19 and disruption of the digital economy; evidence from low and middle-income countries." *Overseas Development Institute* – Digital Pathways at Oxford, Paper Series, Paper 7. Accessed March 14, 2021. https://pathwayscommission.bsg.ox.ac.uk/sites/default/files/2021-01/covid-19_and_disruption_of_the_digital_economy_28jan21.pdf.

Bao, Zhang and Wei Zhao. 2020. "SARS-CoV-2: characteristics and current advances in research." *Virology Journal,* vol. 17, No. 117: 1-17. Accessed 18th January 2021. doi https://doi.org/10.1186/s12985-020-01369-z.

Bearak, Max and Rael Ombuor. 2020. "Police killed at least 20 Kenyans while enforcing coronavirus rules. Hopes for justice are fading." *The Washington Post*, Accessed January 15, 2021. https://www.washingtonpost.com/world/africa/coronavirus-kenya-police-shootings-curfew/2020/12/20/deb81d5a-3efc-11eb-b58b-1623f6267960_story.html.

Bhattacharya, Niranjan and Phillip Stubblefield. 2013. "Of Bioethics, Stem Cells, and Tissue Transplants." In *Human Fetal Tissue Transplantation*. Edited by Niranjan Bhattacharya and Phillip Stubblefield. London: Springer.

Biggs, Brian, Lawrence King, Sanjay Basu and, David Stuckler. 2010. "Is wealthier always healthier? The impact of national income level, inequality, and poverty on public health in Latin America." *Social Science & Medicine*, Vol. 71, No. 2: 266-273. Accessed July 22, 2021. https://doi.org/10.1016/j.socscimed.2010.04.002.

Biryabarema, Elias. 2021. "Kenya Airways says suspends domestic flights after new COVID-19 lockdown announced." *Reuters, Middle East & Africa.* Accessed April 27,

2021. https://www.reuters.com/article/uk-health-coronavirus-kenya-airways-idUSKBN2BJ0CI.

Bogonko, Sorobea Nyachieo. 1985. "Colonial Chiefs and African Development in Kenya with Special Reference To Secular Education." *Transafrican Journal of History* 14: 1-20. Accessed February 10, 2021. http://www.jstor.org/stable/24328515.

Bollyky, Thomas J. and Chad P. Bown. 2020. "The Tragedy of Vaccine Nationalism: Only Cooperation Can End the Pandemic." *Foreign Affairs*, Vol. 99. Accessed October 17, 2020. https://www.foreignaffairs.com/articles/united-states/2020-07-27/vaccine-nationalism-pandemic.

Borra, Surekha. 2020. "COVID-19 Apps: Privacy and Security Concerns." In *Intelligent Systems and Methods to Combat Covid-19*. Edited by A. Joshi, N. Dey and K. Santosh. SpringerBriefs in Applied Sciences and Technology. Springer, Singapore. Accessed February 17, 2021. https://doi.org/10.1007/978-981-15-6572-4_.

Broekaert, Clara, Ceri-Lune Renneboog, Ferdinand Okwaro, Abdu Mohiddin, and Marleen Temmerman. 2021. "Working Paper – Digital News Media Coverage on Sexual and Gender-based Violence in Kenya: Scoping the Impact of the COVID-19 Pandemic." *SocArXiv*. Accessed Jan. 10, 2021. doi:10.31235/osf.io/vbku6.

Broekaert, Clara, Ceri-Lune Renneboog, Ferdinand Okwaro, Abdu Mohiddin, and Marleen Temmerman. 2021. "Working Paper - Digital News Media Coverage on Sexual and Gender-Based Violence in Kenya: Scoping the Impact of the COVID-19 Pandemic." *SocArXiv Papers,* 1-15. Accessed July 24th, 2021. https://ecommons.aku.edu/eastafrica_fhs_mc_obstet_gynaecol/316.

Brooks, John T. and Jay C. Butler. 2021. "Effectiveness of Mask Wearing to Control Community Spread of SARS-CoV-2." *JAMA Insights*. Vol. 325, No. 10: 998-999. Accessed March 10th 2021. doi:10.1001/jama.2021.1505.

Brooks, John T., et al. 2021. "Maximizing Fit for Cloth and Medical Procedure Masks to Improve Performance and Reduce SARS-CoV-2 Transmission and Exposure, 2021." *CDC – Morbidity and Mortality Weekly Report (MMMW)* No. 70: 254–257. Accessed August 7, 2021. doi: http://dx.doi.org/10.15585/mmwr.mm7007e1.

Buguzi, Syriacus. 2021. "Covid-19: Counting the cost of denial in Tanzania." *British Medical Journal*, Vol. 373: n1052. Accessed July 18, 2021. http://dx.doi.org/10.1136/bmj.n1052.

Burlig, Fiona. 2021. *The Impact of Domestic Travel Bans on COVID-19 is Nonlinear in Their Duration.* Washington, DC: NBER.

Callaway, Ewen. 2020. "The coronavirus is mutating — does it matter?" *Nature - News Feature*. Accessed 16 September 2020. https://www.nature.com/articles/d41586-020-02544-6.

Calvin-Smith, Georja and Laura Di Biasio. 2020. "Billionaire Jack Ma's Covid-19 donations to Kenya go missing." *France 24 – Eye on Africa*. Accessed March 9, 2021. https://www.france24.com/en/africa/20200903-kenya-jack-ma-covid-19.

Canudas-Romo, Vladimir. 2018. "Life expectancy and poverty." *The Lancet – Global Health*, Vol. 6: e812. Accessed 3/9/2021. doi: https://doi.org/10.1016/S2214-109X(18)30327-9.

CDC. 2021. "About Variants of the Virus that Causes COVID-19." *National Center for Immunization and Respiratory Diseases (NCIRD), Division of Viral Diseases, The US*

Centers for Disease Control and Prevention. Accessed on June 28, 2021. https://www.cdc.gov/coronavirus/2019-ncov/variants/variant.html.

CDC. 2021. "COVID Data Tracker." *Centers for Disease Control & Prevention*. Accessed July 15th, 2021. https://covid.cdc.gov/covid-data-tracker/#cases_totaltests.

CDC. 2021. "COVID-19: Spread." COVID-19 Frequently Asked Questions." *The Centers for Disease Control and Prevention*. Accessed May 25, 2021. https://www.cdc.gov/coronavirus/2019-ncov/faq.html#Spread.

CDC. 2021. "COVID-19: Understanding mRNA COVID-19 Vaccines." *The US Centers for Disease Control and Prevention*. Accessed Mar. 4, 2021, https://www.cdc.gov/coronavirus/2019-ncov/vaccines/different-vaccines/mrna.html.

CDC. 2020. "Estimated Influenza Illnesses, Medical visits, and Hospitalizations Averted by Vaccination in the United States — 2019–2020 Influenza Season." *Centers for Disease Control and Prevention, National Center for Immunization and Respiratory Diseases (NCIRD).* Accessed May 6, 2021, https://www.cdc.gov/flu/about/burden-averted/2019-2020.htm.

CDC. 2021. "Guidance for Unvaccinated People - Guidance for Wearing Masks." *Centers for Disease Control and Prevention.* Accessed May 19, 2021. https://www.cdc.gov/coronavirus/2019-ncov/prevent-getting-sick/cloth-face-cover-guidance.html.

CDC. 2021. "Polio Vaccination." *Centers for Disease Control and Prevention, National Center for Immunization and Respiratory Diseases (NCIRD).* Accessed May 6, 2021. https://www.cdc.gov/flu/vaccines-work/vaccineeffect.htm.

CDC. 2021. "Science Brief: Community Use of Cloth Masks to Control the Spread of SARS-CoV-2." *Centers for Disease Control and Prevention (CDC).* Accessed July 7th, 2021. https://www.cdc.gov/coronavirus/2019-ncov/science/science-briefs/masking-science-sars-cov2.html.

CDC. 2021. "Vaccine Effectiveness: How Well Do the Flu Vaccines Work? Questions & Answers." *Centers for Disease Control and Prevention, National Center for Immunization and Respiratory Diseases (NCIRD).* Accessed May 6, 2021, https://www.cdc.gov/flu/vaccines-work/vaccineeffect.htm.

CDC. 2020. "What COVID-19 Seroprevalence Surveys Can Tell Us." *Centers for Disease Control and Prevention.* Accessed July 8, 2021, https://www.cdc.gov/coronavirus/2019-ncov/covid-data/seroprevalance-surveys-tell-us.html.

CEIC. 2021. "Kenya Government Debt: % of GDP." *2009 – 2020 CEIC Data.* Accessed May 1, 2021. https://www.ceicdata.com/en/indicator/kenya/government-debt--of-nominal-GDP.

Chakamba, Rumbi. 2021. "Africans view COVID-19 vaccines as less safe than other vaccines." *DEVEX – Inside Development: COVID-19.* Accessed 25th March 2021. https://www.devex.com/news/africans-view-covid-19-vaccines-as-less-safe-than-other-vaccines-99451.

Chandrashekhar, Vaishnavi. 2020. "From leprosy to COVID-19, how stigma makes it harder to fight epidemics." *American Association for the Advancement of Science – Science.* Accessed September 16, 2020. https://www.sciencemag.org/news/2020/09/leprosy-covid-19-how-stigma-makes-it-harder-fight-epidemics.

Chandrashekhar, Vaishnavi.2020. "The burden of stigma." *Science*, Vol. 369, No. 6510: 1419-1423. Accessed 18th September 2020. doi: 10.1126/science.369.6510.1419.

Chaw, Liling, Wee Chian Koh, Sirajul Adli Jamaludin, Lin Naing, Mohammad Fathi Alikhan, and Justin Wong. 2020. "Analysis of SARS-CoV-2 Transmission in Different Settings, Brunei." *Emerging Infectious Diseases*, Vol. 26, No. 11: 2598–2606. Accessed 15th March 2021. doi: 10.3201/eid2611.202263.

Chohan, Usman W. 2021. "Coronavirus and Vaccine Nationalism." *CASS Working Papers on Economics & National Affairs*. Accessed January 16th, 2021. http://dx.doi.org/10.2139/ssrn.3767610.

Chokshi, Dave A. 2018. "Income, Poverty, and Health Inequality." *JAMA*, Vol. 319, No. 13: 1312-1313. Accessed 2nd March 2021. doi:10.1001/jama.2018.2521.

Chukunzira, Angela. 2021. "Organising under curfew: perspectives from Kenya." *Interface: A journal for and about social movements,* Vol. 12, No. 1: 39 – 42. Accessed July 11, 2021. https://www.interfacejournal.net/wp-content/uploads/2020/07/Interface-12-1-Chukunzira.pdf.

CIA. 2021. "Kenya." *The World Factbook*. Accessed June 29, 2021, https://www.cia.gov/the-world-factbook/countries/kenya/.

CIA. 2021. "Tanzania." *The World Factbook*. Accessed June 29, 2021, https://www.cia.gov/the-world-factbook/countries/tanzania/.

Ciekawy, Diane. 1997. "Constitutional and Legal Reform in the Postcolony of Kenya." *Issue: A Journal of Opinion*, Vol. 25, No. 1, (1997), Commentaries in African Studies: Essays about African Social Change and the Meaning of Our Professional Work: 16-18. Accessed 15th May 2021. https://www.jstor.org/stable/1166240.

Citizen Reporter. 2020. "If you fail to wear a mask in public, you risk Ksh.20,000 fine or 6-month jail term." *Citizen Digital*. Accessed May 1, 2020, https://citizentv.co.ke/news/if-you-fail-to-wear-a-mask-in-public-you-risk-ksh-20000-fine-or-six-month-jail-term-329499/.

Coleman, James S. 1990. *Foundations of Social Theory*. Cambridge, MA: Harvard University Press.

Conger, Kate, Jack Healy and Lucy Tompkins. 2010. "Churches Were Eager to Reopen. Now They Are Confronting Coronavirus Cases." *The New York Times,* Accessed July 10, 2021. https://www.nytimes.com/2020/07/08/us/coronavirus-churches-outbreaks.html.

Dahir, A. Latif. 2020. "Kenyans Held for Weeks in Quarantine Were Told to Pay to Get Out." *The New York Times.* Accessed May 8, 2021. https://www.nytimes.com/2020/05/08/world/africa/kenya-coronavirus-quarantine.html.

Daily Nation. 2021. "Kenya's Raila Odinga in isolation after testing positive for Covid-19." *The East African.* Accessed March 12 2021, https://www.theeastafrican.co.ke/tea/news/east-africa/raila-tests-positive-covid-19-3320452.

Danquah, Michael, Simone Schotte, and Kunal Sen. 2020. "COVID-19 and Employment: Insights from the Sub-Saharan African Experience." *Indian Journal of Labor Economics*, Vol. 63: 23–30. Accessed May 7, 2021. https://doi.org/10.1007/s41027-020-00251-4.

Dawa, Jeanette, et al. 2020. "Seasonal influenza vaccination in Kenya: an economic evaluation using dynamic transmission modelling." *BMC Medicine*, Vol. 18, No. 223. Accessed May 8th, 2021. https://doi.org/10.1186/s12916-020-01687-7.

Demeke, Mulat, Josphat Kariuki and Mercy Wanjiru. 2020. "Assessing the Impact of COVID-19 on Food and Nutrition Security and Adequacy of Responses in Kenya." *Food and Agriculture Organization of the United Nations*, Policy Brief.

DeSimone, Daniel C. 2021. "COVID-19 variants: What's the concern?" *Mayo Clinic – Health Information*. Accessed June 17, 2021, https://www.mayoclinic.org/diseases-conditions/coronavirus/expert-answers/covid-variant/faq-20505779.

Dickson, Eva F. Gudgin. *Personal Protective Equipment for Chemical, Biological, and Radiological Hazards: Design, Evaluation and Selection*. Hoboken, NJ: John Wiley & Sons, Inc., 2019.

Doung-ngern, Pawinee et al. 2021. "Associations between Wearing Masks, Washing Hands, and Social Distancing Practices, and Risk of COVID-19 Infection in Public: A Cohort-Based Case-Control Study in Thailand." *SSRN*. Accessed on June 18th, 2020. http://dx.doi.org/10.2139/ssrn.3633162.

Dyer, Owen. 2020. "FGM: nearly 3000 girls are paraded in Kenya as pandemic hinders control efforts." *BMJ: British Medical Journal (Online)*. Vol. 371: m4165. Accessed Oct 28, 2020. doi:10.1136/bmj.m416.

EPA (US). 2021. "EPA Researchers Test Effectiveness of Face Masks, Disinfection Methods Against COVID-19." *United States Environmental Protection Agency*. Accessed on April 5th, 2021. https://www.epa.gov/sciencematters/epa-researchers-test-effectiveness-face-masks-disinfection-methods-against-covid-19.

Equal Measures 2030. 2021. "2019 SDG Gender Index: Key Findings." *Equal Measures 2030 Data Hub*, Accessed on 1st October 2021, https://data.em2030.org/2019-sdg-gender-index/key-findings/.

Equal Measures 2030. 2019. Accessed 2nd March 2021. "Harnessing the Power of Data for Gender Equality – Introducing the 2019 EM2030 SDG Gender Index." *Equal Measures 2030.* URL: https://www.equalmeasures2030.org/wp-content/uploads/2019/07/EM2030_2019_Global_Report_English_WEB.pdf.

Equal Measures 2030. 2021. "SDG Gender Index." *Equal Measures 2030 | Gender Advocates Data Hub, 2021.* Accessed May 16th, 2021. https://www.equalmeasures2030.org/products/sdg-gender-index/.

Escamilla, Veronica, Lisa Calhoun, Norbert Odero and Ilene S. Speizer. 2019. "Access to public transportation and health facilities offering long-acting reversible contraceptives among residents of formal and informal settlements in two cities in Kenya." *Reproductive Health*, Vol. 16, No. 1: 1-22 Accessed May 1, 2021. doi: 10.1186/s12978-019-0828-0.

Evangelist, Cloud. 2019. "Why the least tapped market is the next big thing in cloud." *Cloud Management Insider*, Accessed October 9th, 2020. https://www.cloudmanagementinsider.com/why-african-market-next-big-thing-in-cloud/.

Executive Office of the President (Kenya). 2020. "Executive Order No. 2 of 2020: National Emergency Response Committee on Coronavirus." *The Executive Office of the President: State House – Registry.* Accessed 28th February 2021. https://www.health.go.ke/wp-content/uploads/2020/06/Executive-Order-No-2-of-2020_National-Emergency-Response-Committee-on-Coronavirus-28.2.20.pdf.

FAO, IFAD and WFP. 2015. *The State of Food Insecurity in the World 2015. Meeting the 2015 international hunger targets: taking stock of uneven progress.* Rome: FAO.

Ference, Meghan E. 2021. "'You will build me': fiscal disobedience, reciprocity and the dangerous negotiations of redistribution on Nairobi's matatu." *Africa*. Vol. 91, No. 1: 16-34. Accessed March 3, 2021. doi: https://doi.org/10.1017/S0001972020000820.

Gachane, Ndungu. 2021. "Police arrest man in Mũrang'a after wife claims he forced her to undergo FGM." *The Standard.* Accessed August 3rd 2021. https://www.standardmedia.co.ke/central/article/2001417266/police-arrest-man-in-muranga-after-wife-claims-he-forced-her-to-undergo-fgm.

Gai, Knollyne Oindih and Musa Nyakora. 2020. "Kenya's Leadership Response to Covid-19 Pandemic and Possible Interventions between March and June 2020." *East African Journal of Education and Social Sciences*. Vol. 1, No. 3: 113. Accessed March 24, 2021. doi: https://doi.org/10.46606/eajess2020v01i03.0049.

Ghosh, Nimisha, Indrajit Saha, Jnanendra Prasad Sarkar, and Ujjwal Maulik. 2021. "Strategies for COVID-19 Epidemiological Surveillance in India: Overall Policies till June 2021." *Front Public Health*, 9. Accessed May 2, 2021. doi: 10.3389/fpubh.2021.708224.

GlaxoSmithKline Australia. 2004. "Polio Sabin(TM) (Oral) Multidose: Live Oral Poliomyelitis Vaccine – Consumer Medicine Information Leaflet." GlaxoSmithKline Australia, *CMI Issue #3.* Accessed 5 May 2020. https://apps.medicines.org.au/files/gwcpolin.pdf.

Global Hunger Index. 2020. "Kenya." *Global Hunger Index, 2020.* Accessed 24th March 2021. https://www.globalhungerindex.org/kenya.html.

Gov.UK. 2021. "Foreign travel advice – Kenya." *UK Government.* Accessed 24th March 2021. https://www.gov.uk/foreign-travel-advice/kenya/coronavirus.

Government Printer's Office (GPO). 1950. *The Official Gazette of the Colony and Protectorate of Kenya*, Vol. LII - No. 50. Accessed 24th March 2021. https://gazettes.africa/archive/ke/1950/ke-government-gazette-dated-1950-10-17-no-50.pdf.

Gwenzi, Willis. 2021. "Leaving no stone unturned in light of the COVID-19 faecal-oral hypothesis? A water, sanitation and hygiene (WASH) perspective targeting low-income countries." *Science of The Total Environment*, Vol. 753: 141751. Accessed May 2, 2021. https://doi.org/10.1016/j.scitotenv.2020.141751.

Gygli, Savina, Florian Haelg, Niklas Potrafke and Jan-Egbert Sturm. 2019. "The KOF Globalisation Index – Revisited." *Review of International Organizations,* Vol. 14, No. 3: 543-574 Accessed April 20th, 2021. https://doi.org/10.1007/s11558-019-09344-2.

H.M. Government, UK. 1963. "Statutory Instruments 1963 No. 1968 Kenya: The Kenya Independence Order in Council, 1963." *The Kenya Gazette - Extraordinary Issue – Kenya Gazette Supplement No. 105*, (Legislative Supplement No. 69). Accessed May 1, 2021. http://Kenyalaw.org/kl/fileadmin/pdfdownloads/1963_constitution.pdf.

Hafner, Marco, Erez Yerushalmi, Clement Fays, Eliane Dufresne and Christian van Stolk. 2020. "Practical implications of "vaccine nationalism": A short-sighted and risky approach in response to COVID-19." *RAND Europe, Research Paper* No. 124. Accessed March 24, 2021. http://hdl.handle.net/10419/232250.

Hamann, Ralph, et al. 2020. "COVID-19 in Africa: Contextualizing Impacts, Responses, and Prospects." *Environment: Science and Policy for Sustainable Development*, Vol. 62, No. 6 (Where Do We Go From Here? Reframing Sustainability for a Post-COVID-

19 Era): 8-18. Accessed 24th March 2021. https://doi.org/10.1080/001391 57.2020.1820293.

Harison Lagat, et al. 2020. "Impact of the COVID-19 Pandemic on HIV Testing and Assisted Partner Notification Services, Western Kenya." *AIDS and Behavior*, vol. 24: 3010–3013. Accessed on May 4th, 2021. https://doi.org/10.1007/s10461-020-02938-7.

Harvard Medical School. 2021. "If you've been exposed to the coronavirus." *Harvard Health Publishing* (Harvard Medical School). Accessed July 2, 2021. https://www.health.harvard.edu/diseases-and-conditions/if-youve-been-exposed-to-the-coronavirus.

Haseltine, William A. 2021. "What Are The 677 Mutations? New Covid-19 Variants Found in the US." *Forbes*. Accessed on March 19th, 2021. https://www.forbes.com/sites/williamhaseltine/2021/02/19/what-are-the-677-mutations-new-covid-19-variants-found-in-the-us/.

Hassoun, Nicole. 2021. "Against vaccine nationalism." *Journal of Medical Ethics*. Accessed on 15th March, 2021. http://dx.doi.org/10.1136/medethics-2020-107193.

Hausman, Daniel M. 2021."Philosophy of Economics." *The Stanford Encyclopedia of Philosophy (Spring 2021 Edition)*, Edward N. Zalta (ed.). Accessed May 3, 2021. https://plato.stanford.edu/archives/spr2021/entries/economics/.

Herman, Michael. 2001. *Intelligence Services in the Information Age*. New York: Routledge.

Herskovits, Melville J. 1926. "The Cattle Complex in East Africa." *American Anthropologist*, New Series, Vol. 28, No. 1: 230-272. Accessed May 3, 2021. https://www.jstor.org/stable/660813.

Howard, Jeremy, et al. 2021. "An evidence review of face masks against COVID-19." *Proceedings of the National Academy of Sciences (PNAS)*, Vol. 118, No. 4: e2014564118. Accessed March 24, 2021. doi: 10.1073/pnas.2014564118.

HRW. 2020. "Kenya: Quarantine Conditions Undermine Rights: Ensure Access to Health Care, Sanitation, Information." *Human Rights Watch*. Accessed September 28, 2020. https://www.hrw.org/news/2020/05/28/kenya-quarantine-conditions-undermine-rights.

HRW. 2021. "'We Are All Vulnerable Here': Kenya's Pandemic Cash Transfer Program Riddled With Irregularities." *Human Rights Watch*. Accessed August 20th, 2021. https://www.hrw.org/report/2021/07/20/we-are-all-vulnerable-here/kenyas-pandemic -cash-transfer-program-riddled.

Hu, Ben, Hua Guo, Peng Zhou and Zheng-Li Shi. 2021. "Characteristics of SARS-CoV-2 and COVID-19." *Nature Reviews Microbiology* Vol. 19: 141–154. Accessed June 4, 2021. https://doi.org/10.1038/s41579-020-00459-7.

Huaxia. 2021. "Kenya extends curfew, ramp up vaccination to contain COVID-19." *Xinhua*. Accessed July 30th, 2021. http://www.xinhuanet.com/english/africa/2021-06/30/c_1310034770.htm.

Igunza, Emmanuel. 2020. "Coronavirus corruption in Kenya: Officials and businesspeople targeted." *BBC News*. Accessed 4 May, 2021. https://www.bbc.com/news/world-africa-54278417.

IMF. 2021. "IMF Country Focus: IMF Loan to Support Economic Recovery in Kenya." *The International Monetary Fund.* Accessed April 18, 2021, https://www.imf.org/en/News/Articles/2021/03/17/na031721-imf-loan-to-support-economic-recovery-in-kenya.

International Trade Administration. 2020. "Kenya - Country Commercial Guide: Agribusiness." *International Trade Administration.* Accessed 13th October, 2020. https://www.trade.gov/country-commercial-guides/kenya-agribusiness.

IOM & WFP. 2020."Populations at risk: Implications of COVID-19 for hunger, migration and displacement: An Analysis of Food Security Trends in Major Migration Hotspots." *World Food Programme (WFP) and the International Organization for Migration (IOM).* Accessed January 20, 2021. https://www.iom.int/sites/default/files/populations_at_risk_-_implications_of_covid-19_for_hunger_migration_and_displacement.pdf.

IUCN. 2021. "Kenya - Arid and semi-arid lands." *IUCN, International Union for Conservation of Nature.* Accessed May 4th, 2021. https://www.iucn.org/restoration-initiative/projects/kenya-arid-and-semi-arid-lands.

Jaguga, Florence and Edith Kwobah. 2020. "Mental health response to the COVID-19 pandemic in Kenya: a review." *International Journal of Mental Health Systems*, Vol. 14, No. 68. Accessed March 24th, 2021. https://doi.org/10.1186/s13033-020-00400-8.

Janssens, Wendy, Menno Pradhan, Richard de Groot, Estelle Sidze, Hermann Donfouet, and Amanuel Abajobir. 2020. "The short-term economic effects of COVID-19 and risk-coping strategies of low-income households in Kenya: A rapid analysis using weekly financial household data." *Tinbergen Institute Discussion Paper*, TI 2020-040/V, Tinbergen Institute. Accessed May3, 2021. http://dx.doi.org/10.2139/ssrn.3640340.

John, Neetu, Charlotte Roy, Mary Mwangi, Neha Raval and Terry McGovern. 2021. "COVID-19 and gender-based violence (GBV): hard-to-reach women and girls, services, and programmes in Kenya." *Gender & Development,* Vol. 29, No. 1: 55-71 Gender, development and health. Accessed on September 3rd, 2021. https://doi.org/10.1080/13552074.2021.1885219.

Kagucia, E. Wangeci, et al., 2021. "Seroprevalence of anti-SARS-CoV-2 IgG antibodies among truck drivers and assistants in Kenya," *medXRiv*. Accessed on 7th July, 2021. https://doi.org/10.1101/2021.02.12.21251294.

Kangogo, Janet J. 2020. "The Elements of Drama in Koito a Traditional Wedding Ceremony Among the Tugen People of Baringo Kenya." *CHSS Thesis and Dissertations – UoN Digital Repository.* UoN Research Archive. Accessed May 15th, 2021. http://erepository.uonbi.ac.ke/handle/11295/154605.

Kansiime, Monica K., Justice A. Tambo, Idah Mugambia, Mary Bundi, Augustine Kara, and Charles Owuor. 2021. "COVID-19 implications on household income and food security in Kenya and Uganda: Findings from a rapid assessment." *World Development*, Vol. 137: 2-3. Accessed March 23, 2021.https://doi.org/10.1016/j.worlddev.2020.105199.

Kasuku, Andrew. 2020. "Tables turn: Mob beats up cop after confrontation over a mask." *The Star*. Accessed on 11th November 2020, https://www.the-star.co.ke/news/2020-07-11-mob-beats-up-cop-after-confrontation-over-a-mask/.

Katelaris, Anthea L., et al. 2021. "Epidemiologic Evidence for Airborne Transmission of SARS-CoV-2 during Church Singing, Australia, 2020," *Emerging Infectious Diseases Journal*, Vol. 27, No. 6: 677-1680. Accessed on May 1, 2021. doi:10.3201/eid2706.210465.

Katz, Ingrid T., Rebecca Weintraub, Linda-Gail Bekker, and Allan M. Brandt. 2021. "From Vaccine Nationalism to Vaccine Equity — Finding a Path Forward." *New England Journal of Medicine*, No. 384: 1281-1283. Accessed May 18th, 2021. doi: 10.1056/NEJMp210361.

Kavanagh, Matthew M., et al. 2020. "Access to lifesaving medical resources for African countries: COVID-19 testing and response, ethics, and politics." *Viewpoint*, Vol. 395, No. 10238: 1735-1738. Accessed May 9th, 2021. doi: https://doi.org/10.1016/S0140-6736(20)31093-X.

Kemboi, Leo Kipkogei. 2020. "*Assessment of Kenya's Preparedness for the COVID-19 Emergency*." *SSRN Electronic Journal* Accessed April 27, 2021. http://dx.doi.org/10.2139/ssrn.3609153.

KEMRI & Wellcome Trust. 2020. "Kenya Scientists Release Genome sequencing for the Covid-19 Cases in Kenya." *Kenya Medical Research Institute (KEMRI) & Wellcome Trust.* Accessed June 1st, 2021, https://kemri-wellcome.org/zp-content/uploads/2020/06/Genome-sequencing-of-SARS-CoV-2-cases-in-Kenya.-Report-2-2.pdf.

Kenya Bureau of Standards (KEBS). 2020. "Personal Protective Equipment – Face Masks – Masks for public use – Requirements and Test Method." *Draft Kenya Standard – DKS 2924:2020*. KEBS. Accessed on 5th April, 2021. https://members.wto.org/crnattachments/2020/TBT/KEN/20_4722_00_e.pdf.

Kenya National Assembly. 2009. *Kenya National Assembly Official Record (Hansard).* Nairobi: Government Printing Office.

Kessler, Glenn, Salvador Rizzo and Meg Kelly. 2021. "Trump's false or misleading claims total 30,573 over 4 years." *The Washington Post – Fact Checker*. Accessed March 24, 2021. https://www.washingtonpost.com/politics/2021/01/24/trumps-false-or-misleading-claims-total-30573-over-four-years/.

Khema, Stuti. 2020. "An Opportunity to Build Legitimacy and Trust in Public Institutions in the Time of COVID-19." *World Bank Research & Policy Briefs*, No. 32 – World Bank Malaysia Hub. Accessed May 4, 2021. https://ssrn.com/abstract=3602352.

Kibe, Peter M., Lyagamula Kisia, and Pauline Bakibinga. 2020. "COVID-19 and community healthcare: perspectives from Nairobi's informal settlements." *Pan African Medical Journal*, Vol. 35: 1-3, (Suppl 2): 106. Accessed 25th March 2021. doi: 10.11604/pamj.supp.2020.35.24532.

Kimani, Samuel, Caroline W. Kabiru, Jacinta Muteshi, and Jaldesa Guyo. 2020. "Female genital mutilation/cutting: Emerging factors sustaining medicalization related changes in selected Kenyan communities." *PLOS One*. Accessed 19th March, 2021. https://doi.org/10.1371/journal.pone.0228410.

Kimetto, Kiprotich. 2020. "South African woman quarantined in Nakuru commits suicide." *Citizen Digital*. Accessed March 27, 2021. https://citizentv.co.ke/news/south-african-woman-quarantined-in-nakuru-commits-suicide-328133/.

Kithiia, Justus, Innocent Wanyonyi, Joseph Maina, Titus Jefwa and Majambo Gamoyo. 2020. "The socio-economic impacts of Covid-19 restrictions: Data from the coastal city of Mombasa, Kenya." *Data in Brief*, Vol. 33. Accessed on March 25th, 2021. https://doi.org/10.1016/j.dib.2020.106317.

Kizza, Joseph M. 2003. *Ethical and Social Issues in the Information Age.* 2nd Ed. New York: Springer.

Kotlar, Bethany, Emily Gerson, Sophia Petrillo, Ana Langer and Henning Tiemeier. 2021. "The impact of the COVID-19 pandemic on maternal and perinatal health: a scoping review." *Reproductive Health*, Vol.18, Nol. 10. Accessed 25th March 2021. https://doi.org/10.1186/s12978-021-01070-6.

Kurlander, Carl and Randy P. Juhl. 2020. "Lessons from how the polio vaccine went from the lab to the public that Americans can learn from today." *American Society for Biochemistry and Molecular Biology*. Accessed November 26, 2020. https://www.asbmb.org/asbmb-today/science/092620/lessons-from-how-the-polio-vaccine-went-from-the-l.

La Fontaine, Jean. 2012. "Witchcraft belief is a curse on Africa." *The Guardian – Africa Comment*, Accessed 21st March, 2021, https://www.theguardian.com/commentisfree/belief/2012/mar/01/witchcraft-curse-africa-kristy-bamu.

La Grassa, Jennifer. 2020. "Epidemiologist says small spaces where people spend lots of time have increase transmission risk." *Canadian Broadcasting Corporation News*. Accessed November 31, 2020. https://www.cbc.ca/news/canada/windsor/covid-19-church-spreader-event-1.5783090.

Laiboni, Nkirote. 2020. "Kenya's Philanthropic Tradition Tackles the COVID-19 Challenge." *Coronavirus Response: Chatham House – Expert Comment.* Accessed 9th June 2020. https://www.chathamhouse.org/2020/06/kenyas-philanthropic-tradition-tackles-covid-19-challenge.

Lindsley, William G., Francoise M. Blachere, Brandon F. Law, Donald H. Beezhold and John D. Noti. 2021. "Efficacy of face masks, neck gaiters and face shields for reducing the expulsion of simulated cough-generated aerosols." *Aerosol Science and Technology*, Vol. 55, No. 4: 449-457. Accessed 2 May, 2021. https://doi.org/10.1080/02786826.2020.1862409.

Loewenberg, Sam. 2014. "Breaking the cycle: drought and hunger in Kenya." *The Lancet*, Vol. 383, No. 9922: 1025-1028 (special report). Accessed March 22, 2021. doi: https://doi.org/10.1016/S0140-6736(14)60492-X.

LSSC. 2021. "Dr. Francis Collins Discusses the Complexities of Herd Immunity." *The Late Show with Stephen Colbert*. Accessed on Monday, May 24, 2021. https://web.facebook.com/watch/?extid=SEO----&v=517966956001950.

LSSC. 2021. "Gina Yashere Built Elevators Before Becoming a Comedian." *The Late Show with Stephen Colbert*. Accessed on May 20, 2021. https://web.facebook.com/colbertlateshow/videos/482624979775308/.

Madgavkar, Anu, Olivia White, Mekala Krishnan, Deepa Mahajan, and Xavier Azcue. 2020. "COVID-19 and gender equality: Countering the regressive effects." *McKinsey Global Institute*. Accessed July 1, 2021. https://www.apucis.com/frontend-assets/porto/initial-reports/COVID-19-and-gender-equality-Countering-the-regressive-effects-vF.pdf.pagespeed.ce.DDg-UdcoaA.pdf.

Maeda, Justin M. and John N. Nkengasong. 2021. "The puzzle of the COVID-19 pandemic in Africa." *Science*, Vol. 371, No. 6524: 27-28. Accessed April 21st, 2021. doi: 10.1126/science.abf8832.

Mambo, R. M. 1981. "Local Native Councils and Education in Kenya: The Case of the Coast Province, 1925 to 1950." *Transafrican Journal of History*, Vol. 10, No. 1/2: 61-86. Accessed on 24th March, 2021. https://www.jstor.org/stable/24328588.

Matheka, Duncan Mwangangi, Jolynne Mokaya and Marybeth Maritim. 2013. "Overview of influenza virus infections in Kenya: past, present and future." *The Pan African Medical Journal*, vol. 14, No. 138. Accessed May 1st, 2021. doi: 10.11604/pamj.2013.14.138.2612.

Mbogo, Rachel Waema and John W. Odhiambo. 2021. "COVID-19 outbreak, social distancing and mass testing in Kenya-insights from a mathematical model." *Afrika Matematika*. Accessed April 18th, 2021. https://doi.org/10.1007/s13370-020-00859-1.

Mbula, Ruth. 2020. "Nyamira Governor John Nyangarama dies aged 74." *Business Daily (Africa) – Counties*. Accessed February 18th 2021. https://www.businessdailyafrica.com/bd/news/counties/nyamira-governor-john-nyagarama-dies-aged-74-3232608.

Migrani, Suzi. 2018. "Spectacles of Terror: Media and the Cultural Production of Terrorism." In *Media in the Middle East: Activism, Politics, and Culture*. Edited by Nele Lenze, Charlotte Schriwer and Zubaidah Abdul Jalil. 107-142. New York: Palgrave Macmillan.

Milgram, Stanley. 1967. "The Small World Problem." *Psychology Today*, vol. 1, no. 1: 61-66.

Ministry of Health. 2021. *COVID-19 Update*. Ministry of Health, Republic of Kenya. Accessed 15th July 2021. https://www.health.go.ke/.

Moeen, Muhammad Saad, et al. 2020. *COVID-19: Estimating impact on the economy and poverty in Pakistan: Using the SAM Multiplier Model*. Pakistan: IFPRI/PACE.

Moulin, Emily. 2020. "Nine-Year-Old Kenyan Boy Builds Hand Sanitizing Station to help Fight COVID-19." *Dogonews.com*. Accessed December 10th, 2020. https://www.dogonews.com/2020/8/10/nine-year-old-kenyan-boy-builds-hand-sanitizing-station-to-help-fight-covid-19.

Moyo, Mary-Jean and Tania Lozansky. 2020. "Working with Africa's apparel makers to produce personal protective equipment." *Nasikiliza (World Bank Blogs)*. Accessed May 19, 2021. https://blogs.worldbank.org/nasikiliza/working-africas-apparel-makers-produce-personal-protective-equipment.

Müller, Jürgen D. 1994. "Spanish Influenza in Kenya." *Staff Seminar Paper* No. 6. University of Hannover. Accessed March 24th, 2021. https://www.academia.edu/31804192/Spanish_Influenza_in_Kenya.pdf.

Mulwa, Martin and Timothy Gichana. 2020. "Does education reduce gender differentials in labor market participation? A Kenyan perspective." *African Development Review*. Accessed March 25th, 2021. https://doi.org/10.1111/1467-8268.12451.

Mungai, Allan. 2021. "Report reveals 1.5 million Kenyans are facing hunger as locusts, COVID bites." *Financial Standard*. Accessed February 25th 2021. https://www.standardmedia.co.ke/business/financial-standard/article/2001404502/report-reveals-15million-kenyans-are-facing-hunger.

Murimi, Maureen. 2015. "Bungoma residents protest Kshs. 100,000 wheelbarrows." *Citizen Digital.* Accessed 8th August 2021. https://citizentv.co.ke/news/bungoma-residents-protest-ksh-100000-wheelbarrows-100195/.

Mutahi, Basillioh. 2020. "Coronavirus: The fear of being sentenced to a Kenyan quarantine centre." *BBC News.* Accessed 20 April 2020. https://www.bbc.com/news/world-africa-52326316.

Mutahi, Patrick and Kate Jane Wanjiru. 2020. "Police Brutality and Solidarity during the COVID-19 Pandemic in Mathare." *Mambo!* Vol. XVII, no. 6. Accessed March 24th, 2021. https://mambo.hypotheses.org/2895. ffhalshs-03078529.

Nakkazi, Esther. 2020. "Obstacles to COVID-19 control in East Africa." *Lancet Infectious Diseases*, Vol. 20, No. 6: 660. Accessed March 4th, 2021. doi: 10.1016/S1473-3099(20)30382-0.

Namu, John-Allan and Tess Riley. "Nine weeks of bloodshed: how brutal policing of Kenya's Covid curfew left 15 dead." 2020. *The Guardian/Global Development/Human Rights in Focus*. Accessed 23rd December 2020. https://www.theguardian.com/global-development/2020/oct/23/brutal-policing-kenyas-covid-curfew-left-15-dead.

National Council for Law Reporting 2009. "Laws of Kenya – The Public Order Act, Chapter 56," *Kenya Law Reports – National Council for Law Reporting/Attorney General, 2003* (rev. 2009). Accessed March 24th, 2021. http://www.kenyalaw.org.

National Council for Law Reporting "Laws of Kenya: The Chiefs' Act, Chapter 128," *Kenya Law Reports – National Council for Law Reporting, 1998* (rev. 2012), http://extwprlegs1.fao.org/docs/pdf/ken102000.pdf.

Nature Editors. 2021. "To curb COVID-19, global health must go local." *Nature Medicine*, Vol. 27, No. 929. Accessed March 4th, 2021. https://doi.org/10.1038/s41591-021-01400-y.

Nechifor, V., E. Ferrari, E. Kihiu, J. Laichena, D. Omanyo, R. Musamali and B. Kiriga. 2020. *COVID-19 impacts and short-term economic recovery in Kenya.* EUR 30296 EN, Publications Office of the EU, Luxembourg, 2020, doi:10.2760/767447, JRC121284.

Neetu John, Charlotte Roy, Mary Mwangi, Neha Raval and Terry McGovern. 2021. "COVID-19 and gender-based violence (GBV): hard-to-reach women and girls, services, and programmes in Kenya." *Gender & Development*, Vol. 29, No. 1: 55-71. Accessed May 24th, 2021. doi: 10.1080/13552074.2021.1885219.

NERC. 2021. "Update on COVID-19 in the Country and Response Measures, as at April 22, 2021." Day 402, Brief No. 394 (Press Statements). *Ministry of Health's National Emergency Response Committee.* Accessed May 1, 2021. https://www.health.go.ke/wp-content/uploads/2021/04/NERC-MOH-CS-COVID-UPDATE-22.4.2021.pdf.

Ngugi, Brian. 2021. "Matiang'i extends night curfew by 60 days to curb Covid-19 spread." *Business Daily – Economy.* Accessed May 31 2021. https://www.business dailyafrica.com/bd/economy/matiang-i-extends-night-curfew-by-60-days--3419762.

Ngwacho, Areba George. 2021. "COVID-19 Pandemic Impact on Kenyan Education Sector: Learner Challenges and Mitigations." *Journal of Research Innovation and Implications in Education*, Vol. 4, No. 2: 128-139. Accessed March 24th, 2021. https://jriiejournal.com/wp-content/uploads/2021/03/JRIIE-4-2-015.pdf.

Nhemachena, Artwell, Nelson Mlambo and Maria Kaundjua. 2016. "The Notion of the 'Field' and the Practices of Researching and Writing Africa: Towards Decolonial Praxis." *Africology: The Journal of Pan African Studies*, vol. 9, no. 7: 15-36.

Noreh, A. V. 1968. "Harambee in Kenya: A Bibliography." University of Nairobi Library. Accessed on 20th December, 2020. http://erepository.uonbi.ac.ke/bitstream/handle/11295/40009/Norey%20A.%20V.pdf?sequence=1.

NTV Kenya. 2021. *NTV Kenya Facebook.* Accessed March 24th, 2021. http://ow.ly.kiZP50yQTIj.

OCHA Services. 2021. "Total COVID-19 Tests Performed by Country." *Humanitarian Data Exchange* (HDX). Accessed on May 29th, 2021. https://data.humdata.org/dataset/total-covid-19-tests-performed-by-country.

O'Dowd, Adrian. 2021."Covid-19: Cases of delta variant rise by 79%, but rate of growth slows." *The British Medical Journal*, Vol. 373. Accessed March 23rd, 2021. doi: https://doi.org/10.1136/bmj.n1596.

Ojwang', Frank. 2021. "Human Rights Violations During COVID-19 Curfew in Kenya: When Poverty Increases Chances of Preventable Death." In *Governing the Crisis: Law, Human Rights and COVID-19*. 203-31. Edited by Stefan Kirchner. Zürich: LIT Verlag.

Okal, Benard O., Benard O. Kodak, Adams Yakub and Jackline Okello. 2020. "Implications of Coronavirus (Covid-19) on the Stability of the Luo Cultural Funeral Ceremonies in Kenya." *EAS Journal of Humanities and Cultural Studies*, Vol. 2, No. 2: 96-103. Accessed March 3, 2021. doi:10.36349/EASJHCS.2020.V02I02.015.

Okuku, Eric, et al. 2021. "The impacts of COVID-19 pandemic on marine litter pollution along the Kenyan Coast: A synthesis after 100 days following the first reported case in Kenya." *Marine Pollution Bulletin*, Vol. 162. Accessed on 15th May, 2021. https://doi.org/10.1016/j.marpolbul.2020.111840.

Ole Masago, Morompi, Bakari Chaka, Kelele Joshua, Sambu Alice, Jebet Sheila, and G. Reuben. 2020. "Effects of Covid-19 Pandemic on the Welfare of the Maasai Girl Child in Narok County, Kenya." *European Journal of Social Sciences*, Vol. 2020, Vol. 3, No. 3: 123 – 132. Accessed April 15th, 2021. http://hdl.handle.net/123456789/11071.

Ornstein, Charles and Ash Ngu. 2020. "No, President Trump, Testing Is Not Causing Case Counts to Rise. The Virus Is Just Spreading Faster." *ProPublica – Coronavirus*. Accessed on June 25, 2021. https://www.propublica.org/article/state-coronavirus-data-doesnt-support-trumps-misleading-testing-claims.

OSAC. 2021. "Health Alert: Dar es Salaam (Tanzania), Change in Entry Requirements Due to COVID-19." *Overseas Security Advisory Council, Bureau of Diplomatic Security, U.S. Department of State*. Accessed 5th May, 2021. https://www.osac.gov/Content/Report/0b5edea9-2158-43e5-a2b6-1b83766efd6b.

Oudia, Rushdie. 2021. "Kenya: Nyanza, Western Counties Brace for the Worst of Covid-19 Wave." *Daily Nation*. Accessed June 29th, 2021. https://nation.africa/kenya/counties/nyanza-western-brace-for-the-worst-of-covid-wave-3430592.

Ouma, Polet Njeri, Abednego Nzyuko Masai, and Israel Nyaburi Nyadera. 2020. "Health coverage and what Kenya can learn from the COVID-19 pandemic." *Journal of Global Health*, vol. 10: 362. Accessed 14th April 2021. doi: 10.7189/jogh.10.020362.

Ouma, Samuel. "COVID-19: Are Destitute Kenyans Sharing Masks?" *Pan African Visions.* Accessed April 14, 2021. https://panafricanvisions.com/2020/04/covid-19are-destitute-kenyans-sharing-masks/0000.

Ourworldindata. 2017. "Corruption Perception Index vs. Share of people who have bribed, 2017." *Our World in Data.* Accessed 7/28/2021. https://ourworldindata.org/grapher/share-of-people-paying-bribes-vs-corruption-perception.

Ourworldindata. 2017. "Perception of Corruption by Institution, World, 2017." *Our World In Data.* Accessed July 28th, 2021. https://ourworldindata.org/grapher/perception-of-corruption-by-institution?country.

Ourworldindata. 2013. "Average rating of perceived corruption in public sector, 2013." *Our World in Data.* Accessed July 28, 2021. https://ourworldindata.org/grapher/average-rating-of-corruption-perception.

Owino, Boniface. 2020 "Kenya's Covid-19 budget: Funding for health and welfare." *Development Initiatives.* Accessed 2 July 2020. https://devinit.org/resources/kenyas-covid-19-budget-funding-for-health-and-welfare/.

Pallangyo, Eunice, Mary Grace Nakate, Rose Maina, and Valerie Fleming. 2020. "The impact of covid-19 on midwives' practice in Kenya, Uganda and Tanzania: A reflective account." *Midwifery*, 89: 102775. Accessed 14th April 2021. doi: 10.1016/j.midw.2020.102775.

Pardi, Norbert, Michael J. Hogan, Frederick W. Porter and Drew Weissman. 2018. "mRNA vaccines — a new era in vaccinology." *Nature Reviews Drug Discovery,* vol. 17: 261–279. Accessed 14th April 2021. https://doi.org/10.1038/nrd.2017.243.

Paz, Christian. 2020. "All the President's Lies About the Coronavirus." *The Atlantic – Politics.* Accessed May 1, 2021. https://www.theatlantic.com/politics/archive/2020/11/trumps-lies-about-coronavirus/608647/.

Peralta, Eyder. 2020. "In Kenya, Security Forces Attack Ferry Passengers Trying To Make Coronavirus Curfew." *NPR – The Coronavirus Crisis.* Accessed March 27, 2021. https://www.npr.org/sections/coronavirus-live-updates/2020/03/27/822559 830/in-kenya-security-forces-attack-ferry-passengers-trying-to-make-coronavirus-curf.

Phelan, Alexandra L., Mark Eccleston-Turner, Michelle Rourke, Allan Maleche, and Chenguang Wang. 2020. "Legal agreements: barriers and enablers to global equitable COVID-19 vaccine access." *The Lancet*, vol. 396, no. 10254: 800. Accessed 17th April 2021. https://doi.org/10.1016/S0140-6736(20)31873-0.

Presidential Strategic Communication Unit (PSCU). 2020. *Address to the Nation by H.E. Uhuru Kenyatta on Covid-19 [...]* Accessed 15th March 2021. URL: https://www.president.go.ke/2020/03/15/.

Presidential Strategic Communication Unit (PSCU). 2021. *The Fourteenth [14th] Presidential Address on the Coronavirus Pandemic.* Accessed 12th May, 2021. https://www.president.go.ke/2021/03/12.

PSCU. 2020. "Governor Nyangarama was a True Servant Leader, President Kenyatta Says." *Presidential Strategic Communications Unit.* State House. Accessed December 18th, 2020. https://www.president.go.ke/2020/12/18/governor-nyagarama-was-a-true-servant-leader-president-kenyatta-says/.

PSCU. 2021. "President Kenyatta Mourns Kiambaa MP Paul Koinange." *Presidential Strategic Communications Unit.* State House. Accessed May 31, 2021. https://www.president.go.ke/2021/03/31/president-kenyatta-mourns-kiambaa-mp-paul-koinange/.

PSCU. 2021. "The Fifteenth [15th] Presidential Address on the Coronavirus Pandemic." *The Presidential Strategic Communications Unit (PSCU).* Accessed May 26th 2021. http://ke.china-embassy.org/chn/lsfw/P020210328027906621415.pdf.

PSCU. 2021. "The Seventh Presidential Address on the Coronavirus Pandemic: The 8-Point Economic Stimulus Programme." *PSCU – State House.* Accessed 23rd June 2021. https://www.president.go.ke/2020/05/23/the-seventh-presidential-address-on-the-coronavirus-pandemic-the-8-point-economic-stimulus-programme-saturday-23rd-may-2020/.

PSCU. 2020. "Address to the Nation by H.E. Uhuru Kenyatta […] on Covid-19, Commonly Known as Coronavirus at Harambee House, Nairobi." *The Briefing Room – the Presidency.* Accessed on 25th March 2021. https://www.president.go.ke/2020/03/15/address-to-the-nation-by-h-e-uhuru-kenyatta-c-g-h-president-of-the-republic-of-kenya-and-commander-in-chief-of-the-defence-forces-on-covid-19-commonly-known-as-coronavirus/.

PSCU. 2020. "Address to the Nation on Covid-19, Commonly Known as Coronavirus at Harambee House, Nairobi." *The Briefing Room – the Presidency.* Accessed on 15th March 2021.

PSCU. 2020. "Presidential Address on the State Interventions to Cushion Kenyans against Economic Effects of Covid-19 Pandemic." *The Presidency – Briefing Room (Latest News).* Accessed 25th March, 2021. https://www.president.go.ke/2020/03/25/presidential-address-on-the-state-interventions-to-cushion-kenyans-against-economic-effects-of-covid-19-pandemic-on-25th-march-2020/.

Quaglio, G. L., W. Preiser and G. Putoto. 2020. "COVID-19 in Africa." *Public Health*, vol. 180: 60. Accessed 4th April 2021. doi: 10.1016/j.puhe.2020.05.030.

Quaife, Matthew, et al. 2020. "The impact of COVID-19 control measures on social contacts and transmission in Kenyan informal settlements." *BMC Medicine*, Vol. 18, No. 316. Accessed 14th April 2021. https://doi.org/10.1186/s12916-020-01779-4.

Radhakrishnan, Nita and Devendra Kumar Gupta. 2021. "India's COVID-19 response: science first." *The Lancet – Correspondence*, Vol. 397, No. 10293: 2464-2465. Accessed July 26, 2021. doi: https://doi.org/10.1016/S0140-6736(21)01241-1.

Rafaeli, Tal and Geraldine Hutchinson. 2020. "The Secondary Impacts of COVID-19 on Women and Girls in Sub-Saharan Africa." *K4D Helpdesk Report 830*. Brighton, UK: Institute of Development Studies.

Reardon, Sara. 2021. "The Most Worrying Mutations in Five Emerging Coronavirus Variants." *Scientific American – Public Health.* Accessed on April 29, 2021. https://www.scientificamerican.com/article/the-most-worrying-mutations-in-five-emerging-coronavirus-variants/.

Republic of Kenya. 2013. "Kenya Population Situation Analysis." *National Council for Population and Development (NCPD) and the United Nations Population Fund (UNFPA).* Nairobi. Accessed 14th April 2021. https://www.unfpa.org/sites/default/files/admin-resource/FINALPSAREPORT_0.pdf.

Republic of Kenya (Government Printer). 2017. "The Environmental Management and Co-Ordination Act." *The Kenya Gazette – Special Issue*" *Gazette Notice* No. 2334, Vol. CXIX, No. 31. Accessed 14th March, 2021. https://www.nema.go.ke/images/Docs/Awarness%20Materials/Gazette_legal_Notice_on_carrier_bags.pdf.

Reuters Staff. 2021. "Kenya extends COVID-19 curfew by 60 days." *Reuters*. Accessed May 30, 2021. https://www.reuters.com/article/health-coronavirus-kenya-idUSL5N2NH072.

Ritchie, Hannah, et al. 2021. "Coronavirus (COVID-19) Testing." *Our World in Data*. Accessed April 9, 2021. URL: https://ourworldindata.org/coronavirus-testing#how-many-tests-are-performed-each-day.

Roelen, K., Caroline Ackley, Paul Boyce, Nicolas Farina and Santiago Ripoll. 2020. "COVID-19 in LMICs: The Need to Place Stigma Front and Centre to Its Response." *The European Journal of Development Research,* No. 32: 1592–1612. Accessed 24th April 2021. https://doi.org/10.1057/s41287-020-00316-6.

Roser, Max and Hannah Ritchie. 2019. "Hunger and Undernourishment." *OurWorldInData.org*. Accessed 5th May, 2021. https://ourworldindata.org/hunger-and-undernourishment.

Saleh, Musa. "Impact of COVID-19 on Tanzania Political Economy." *International Journal of Advanced Studies in Social Science & Innovation (IJASSI),* Vol. 4, No. 1 (2020), 24-36, http://dx.doi.org/10.30690/ijassi.41.03.

Sambu, Alice, Kweingoti Reuben, Cherotich Mary Gabriel, and Abdalla Hamadi Salimin. 2021. "Effects of Covid-19 Pandemic on Religious Activities and Faith of Worshippers in Kenya; A Case Study of Narok Town, Kenya." *Journal of Studies in Social Sciences*, Vol. 20: 1-18.

Schmelz, Katrin. 2021. "Enforcement may crowd out voluntary support for COVID-19 policies, especially where trust in government is weak and in a liberal society." *Proceedings of the National Academy of Sciences of the United States of America (PNAS)*, vol. 118, no. 1. Accessed April 5th, 2021. https://doi.org/10.1073/pnas.2016385118.

Sickbert-Bennett, Emily E., et al. 2021. "Fitted Filtration Efficiency of Double Masking During the COVID-19 Pandemic." *JAMA Internal Medicine – Research Letter*. Accessed April 26, 2021. doi:10.1001/jamainternmed.2021.2033.

Songok, Elijah. 2020. "A locally sustainable approach to COVID-19 testing in Africa." *The Lancet Microbe*. Accessed 14th April 2021. doi: https://doi.org/10.1016/S2666-5247(20)30118-X.

Sridhar, S., P. Gautret and P. Brouqui. 2015. "A comprehensive review of the Kumbh Mela: identifying risks for spread of infectious diseases." *Clinical Microbiology and Infection,* Vol. 21, No. 2: 128-133. Accessed 4th April 2021. https://doi.org/10.1016/j.cmi.2014.11.021.

Steingrüber, Sarah, Monica Kirya, David Jackson and Saul Mullard. 2020. "Corruption in the time ofCOVID-19: A double-threat for low income countries." *U4 Brief*, No. 6. Chr. Michelsen Institute. Accessed 19 May 2021. https://www.u4.no/publications/corruption-in-the-time-of-covid-19-a-double-threat-for-low-income-countries.pdf.

Stevens, Laura M., et al. 2021. "Children's Vulnerability to Sexual Violence During COVID-19 in Kenya: Recommendations for the Future." *Frontiers in Global Women's*

Health, Vol. 2: 1-5. Accessed 24th March 2021. https://doi.org/10.3389/fgwh.2021.630901.

Stover, John, et al. "The Risks and Benefits of Providing HIV Services during the COVID-19 Pandemic." 1-11 *MedRxiv*. Accessed March 1, 2021. https://doi.org/10.1101/2021.03.01.21252663.

The Cleveland Clinic. 2021. "What to Know About the Latest COVID-19 Variant and Other Coronavirus Mutations." *Cleveland Clinic – Health Essentials*. Accessed June 22, 2021. https://health.clevelandclinic.org/what-does-it-mean-that-the-coronavirus-is-mutating/.

The Global Economy.com. 2021. "Kenya: Overall globalization." *The Global Economy.Com*. Accessed July 4th, 2021. https://www.theglobaleconomy.com/Kenya/kof_overall_glob/.

The World Bank. 2019. "Kenya Economic Update: Transforming Agricultural Productivity to Achieve Food Security for All." *The World Bank Group – IBRD & IDA*. Accessed April 1, 2021. https://www.worldbank.org/en/country/kenya/publication/kenya-economic-update-transforming-agricultural-productivity-to-achieve-food-security-for-all.

The World Bank. 2018. "Kenya National Electrification Strategy: Key Highlights." *The World Bank Group*. Accessed 31st December 2020. https://pubdocs.worldbank.org/en/413001554284496731/Kenya-National-Electrification-Strategy-KNES-Key-Highlights-2018.pdf.

The World Bank. 2020. *World Bank Approves $1 Billion Financing for Kenya, to Address COVID-19 Financing Gap and Support Kenya's Economy.* The World Bank, Press Release, Accessed May 20, 2021. URL: https://www.worldbank.org/en/news/press-release/2020/05/20/world-bank-approves-1-billion-financing-for-kenya-to-address-covid-19-financing-gap-and-support-kenyas-economy.

Thiga, J. M. 2021. "Impact of COVID-19 Pandemic on the Church's Socioeconomic Well-Being: A Case of Worldwide Gospel Church of Kenya-Githurai Presbytery." I*mpact: Journal of Transformation*, vol. 4, no. 1: 36-45. Accessed 24th June 2021. https://journals.aiu.ac.ke/index.php/impact/article/view/84.

ThinkWell Strategic Purchasing for Primary Health Care. 2020. "COVID-19 Summary Update for Kenya." Washington, DC: ThinkWell, 2020.

TI Kenya. 2020. "Corruption Perception Index 2019." *Corruption Perception Index*. Accessed on 23rd January 2021. https://tikenya.org/corruption-perceptions-index-2019/.

Timmis, Hannah. 2021. "Jobs in Kenya: Opportunities and Challenges." *K4D Helpdesk Report*. Brighton, UK: Institute of Development Studies. Accessed 24th March 2021. https://opendocs.ids.ac.uk/opendocs/handle/20.500.12413/13619.

Transparency International. 2021. "Corruption Perceptions Index." *Transparency International.* Accessed 24th March 2021. https://www.transparency.org/en/cpi/2020/table/ken#.

Umar, Saidu Mohammed, Musa Saleh, Aliyu Mohammed Malami and Nafiu Mahmood Alhaji. 2020. "Politics of Coronavirus in Africa: An Analysis of Kenya and Nigeria." *IJARIIE*, Vol. 6 No. 3. Accessed 24th March 2021. https://d1wqtxts1xzle7.cloudfront.net/64046395.

Umuhoza, Therese, Wallace D. Bulimo, Julius Oyugi, David Schnabel and James D. Mancuso. 2020. "Prevalence and factors influencing the distribution of influenza viruses in Kenya: Seven-year hospital-based surveillance of influenza-like illness (2007–2013)." *PLOS One*. Accessed May 21st 2021. https://doi.org/10.1371/journal.pone.0237857.

UN Habitat. 2021. "Hand washing stations in Nairobi's biggest dumpsite officially launched to tackle COVID-19 pandemic." Accessed on 9th March, 2021. https://unhabitat.org/hand-washing-stations-in-nairobi%E2%80%99s-biggest-dumpsite-officially-launched-to-tackle-covid-19-pandemic.

UNDP. 2020. "Gender Inequality Index." *Human Development Indices: A statistical update 2019 | United Nations Development Programme | UN Data*. Accessed 24th March 2021. http://data.un.org/DocumentData.aspx?id=415.

UNDP. 2021. "Human Development Reports – Gender Inequality Index, 2019." *United Nations Development Program*. Accessed 24th March 2021. URL: http://hdr.undp.org/en/composite/GII.

UNEP. 2021. "Kenya," *UN Environment Programme*. Accessed 25th March 2021. https://www.unep.org/explore-topics/transport/what-we-do/share-road/kenya.

UNFPA. 2020. "Female genital mutilation (FGM) frequently asked questions." *United Nations Population Fund*. Accessed on July 30th, 2021. https://www.unfpa.org/resources/female-genital-mutilation-fgm-frequently-asked-questions.

UNICEF Kenya. 2021. "Water, Sanitation and Hygiene: Improving children's access to water, sanitation and hygiene." *UNICEF – Kenya*. Accessed July 31st, 2021, https://www.unicef.org/kenya/water-sanitation-and-hygiene.

UNICEF. 2020. "A Profile of Female Genital Mutilation in Kenya," *UNICEF*. http://data.unicef.org/wp-content/Fuploads/Profile-of-FGM-in-Kenya-English_2020.pdf.

United Nations. 2004. *The International covenant on civil and political rights (CCPR)*. CCPR/C/KEN/2004/227. New York: United Nations – Human Rights: OHCR.

USAID. 2021. "Kenya: Agriculture and Food Security – Overview." *USAID*. Accessed June 03, 2021. https://www.usaid.gov/kenya/agriculture-and-food-security.

Vaishya, Raju. 2021. "The havoc caused by the second wave of COVID-19 in India." *Apollo Medicine* 0;0:0. Accessed on 28 June, 2021. doi: 10.4103/am.am_36_21.

Velázquez, Francisco R. 2021. "Coronavirus Mutations and Variants: What Does It Mean?" *Spokane Regional Health District (SRHD)*. Accessed April 1st, 2021. https://srhd.org/news/2021/coronavirus-mutations-and-variants-what-does-it-mean.

Villegas, Cirenia Chavez, Silvia Peirolo, Matilde Rocca, Alessandra Ipince, Shivit Bakrania. 2021. "Impacts of health-related school closures on child protection outcomes: A review of evidence from past pandemics and epidemics and lessons learned for COVID-19." *International Journal of Educational Development*, Vol. 84. Accessed May 19, 2021. https://doi.org/10.1016/j.ijedudev.2021.102431.

Wafula, Paul. 2021. "At long last, faces of Covid-19 millionaires start emerging." *Nation Media Group*. Accessed November 24, 2020. https://nation.africa/kenya/news/at-long-last-faces-of-covid-19-millionaires-start-emerging--3208076?view=htmlamp.

Waithera, Alice. 2021. "Men held me down, forcibly cut me - Mũrang'a woman." *The Star – News*, Accessed 6th July 2021. https://www.the-star.co.ke/news/2021-07-05-men-held-me-down-forcibly-cut-me-muranga-woman/.

Wamai, E. Njoki.2014." Mediating Kenya's post-election violence: from a peace-making to a constitutional moment," In *Kenya: The Struggle for a New Constitutional Order*. Edited by Godwin R. Murunga, Dunkan Okelo and Anders Sjogren. London: Zed Books.

Wamsley, Laurel. 2020. "Vatican OKs Receiving COVID-19 Vaccines, Even If Research Involved Fetal Tissue." *NPR – The Coronavirus Crisis – Coronavirus Updates.* Accessed December 21, 2020. https://www.npr.org/sections/coronavirus-live-updates/2020/12/21/948806643/vatican-oks-receiving-covid-19-vaccines-even-if-research-involved-fetal-tissue.

Wangmo, Tenzin. 2020. "Kenya Stops Abusive Forced Quarantine Related to Covid-19: Officials Launch Guidelines for Self-Isolation of Covid-19 Patients." *Human Rights Watch.* Accessed July 31st, 2020 https://www.hrw.org/news/2020/07/31/kenya-stops-abusive-forced-quarantine-related-covid-19.

Watts, Duncan J. 2004. *Six Degrees: The Science of a Connected Age*. New York: W. W. Norton.

Were, Maureen. 2020. "COVID-19 and socioeconomic impact in Africa: The case of Kenya." *UNU-WIDER, WIDER Background Note* 3/2020. Helsinki: UNU-WIDER.

Wheelock, David. 2020. "What Can We Learn from the Spanish Flu Pandemic of 1918-19 for COVID-19?" *Federal Reserve Bank of St. Louis.* Accessed June 1st, 2021. https://www.stlouisfed.org/on-the-economy/2020/june/what-can-we-learn-from-the-spanish-flu-pandemic-of-1918-for-covid-19.

WHO Africa. 2021. "Coronavirus (COVID-19)." *World Health Organization*. Accessed July 16th, 2021. https://www.afro.who.int/health-topics/coronavirus-covid-190.

WHO. 2020. "Coronavirus disease (COVID-19) advice for the public: When and how to use masks." *World Health Organization: Home/Diseases/Coronavirus disease (COVID-19).* Accessed on 1st December, 2020. https://www.who.int/emergencies/diseases/novel-coronavirus-2019/advice-for-public/when-and-how-to-use-masks.

WHO. 2020. "Coronavirus disease (COVID-19): How is it transmitted?" WHO *Q&A – Coronavirus Disease (COVID-19).* Accessed on 13 December 2020. https://www.who.int/news-room/q-a-detail/coronavirus-disease-covid-19-how-is-it-transmitted.

WHO. 2021. "Disability-adjusted life years (DALYs)." *WHO Global Health Observatory*. Accessed July 14th 2021, https://www.who.int/data/gho/indicator-metadata-registry/imr-details/158.

WHO. 2021. "Genome sequencing central to COVID-19 response." *WHO-Regional Office for Africa*. Accessed 25th February 2021. https://www.afro.who.int/news/genome-sequencing-central-covid-19-response.

WHO. 2020. "Novel Coronavirus(2019-nCoV): Situation Report – 10." *The World Health Organization*. Accessed 30th January, 2021. https://www.who.int/docs/default-source/coronaviruse/situation-reports/20200130-sitrep-10-ncov.pdf?sfvrsn=d0b2e 480_2.

WHO. 2020. "Transmission of SARS-CoV-2: implications for infection prevention precautions." *Scientific Brief.* Accessed on 9 July 2021. https://www.who.int/news-room/commentaries/detail/transmission-of-sars-cov-2-implications-for-infection-prevention-precautions.

Wild-Wood, Emma Liz, et al. 2021. "The Public Role of Churches in Early Responses to COVID-19 in Africa: Snapshots from Nigeria, Congo, Kenya and South Africa." *Studies in World Christianity,* Vol. 27, No. 1: 65-84. Accessed 30 March, 2021. https://www.euppublishing.com/doi/abs/10.3366/swc.2021.0326.

Williams, Sarah, Adam White, Peter Waiganjo, Daniel Orwa and Jacqueline Klopp. 2015. "The digital matatu project: Using cell phones to create an open source data for Nairobi's semi-formal bus system." *Journal of Transport Geography,* Vol. 49: 39-51. Accessed February 27, 2021. https://doi.org/10.1016/j.jtrangeo.2015.10.005.

Workie, Endashaw, Joby Mackolil, Joan Nyika and Sendhil Ramadas. 2020. "Deciphering the impact of COVID-19 pandemic on food security, agriculture, and livelihoods: A review of the evidence from developing countries." *Current Research in Environmental Sustainability*, Vol. 2. Accessed May 1, 2021. https://doi.org/10.1016/j.crsust.2020.100014.

World Bank Group. 2021. "Kenya Secures $130 Million for COVID-19 Vaccines." *The World Bank.* Press Release. Accessed June 28, 2021, https://www.worldbank.org/en/news/press-release/2021/06/28/kenya-secures-130-million-for-covid-19-vaccines.

World Economic Forum. *Global Gender Gap Report 2020.* Geneva: The World Economic Forum, 2019. URL: http://www3.weforum.org/docs/WEF_GGGR_2020.pdf.

World Economic Forum. 2021. *Measuring the Global Gender Gap.* Geneva: The World Economic Forum. Accessed 15th March, 2021. https://reports.weforum.org/global-gender-gap-report-2018/measuring-the-global-gender-gap/?doing_wp_cron=1629014648.4019539356231689453125.

World Food Program USA. 2021. "Women are hungrier." *World Food Program USA.* Accessed May 3, 2021. https://www.wfpusa.org/women-are-hungrier-infographic/.

World Hunger. 2020. "Women and Hunger Facts." *World Hunger Education Service.* Accessed on 8th July 2021. https://www.worldhunger.org/women-and-hunger-facts/.

Yitambe, Andre, James Okello, C. M. Ooko Nguka, Caroline Ochieng and Ana Peña del Valle. 2009. "Road Traffic Accidents as an Everyday Hazard: Kisii and Kisumu, Kenya." In *Disaster Risk Reduction: Cases from Urban Africa.* Edited by Mark Pelling and Ben Wisner. New York: Routledge.

Yusuf, Mohammed. 2020. "COVID-19 Pandemic: Kenyans Confined at Quarantine Facilities See It as Sentence." *VOA News.* Accessed May 22, 2021. https://www.voanews.com/covid-19-pandemic/kenyans-confined-quarantine-facilities-see-it-sentence.

Zhiang, Yu. 2016. "The personalized and Personal 'Mass' Media – From 'We-Broadcast' to 'We-Chat': Reflection on the case of Bi Fujian Incident." In *Defining Identity and the Changing Scope of Culture in the Digital Age.* Edited by Alison Novak. Hershey, PA: IGI Global.

Zyskind, Israel, et al. 2021. "SARS-CoV-2 Seroprevalence and Symptom Onset in Culturally Linked Orthodox Jewish Communities across Multiple Regions in the United States." *JAMA Network Open*, Vol. 4, No. 3: e212816. Accessed on May 5th, 2021. doi:10.1001/jamanetworkopen.2021.2816.

Author's Contact Information

Stephen M. Magu, PhD
Assistant Professor of Political Science
Department of Political Science
Norfolk State University
Norfolk, VA USA
Email: smmagu@nsu.edu

Stephen is an avid student (and teacher) of world history, including its several near-extinction calamities, pandemics, conflicts and wars; its responses, reconstruction and foresight before 'the next one.' He researches global political economy, human rights, foreign policy and their intersections in the age of globalization under complex interactions, and within sovereignty and national identity frameworks.

Index

F

G

H

I

K

L

M

N